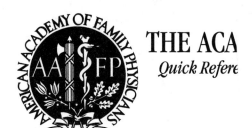

THE ACA

Quick Refere

MW00911786

Children's
Health

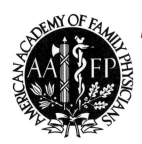

THE ACADEMY COLLECTION
Quick Reference Guides for Family Physicians

Children's Health

JEANNE P. SPENCER, MD

Associate Director
Family Medical Center
Johnstown, Pennsylvania

With

Orlando F. Mills, MD
Program Director
Family Medical Center
Johnstown, Pennsylvania

Series Medical Editor
Richard Sadovsky, MD, MS
Associate Professor of Family Medicine
State University of New York Health Science Center
Brooklyn, New York

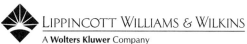

LIPPINCOTT WILLIAMS & WILKINS
A **Wolters Kluwer** Company

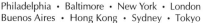

Philadelphia · Baltimore · New York · London
Buenos Aires · Hong Kong · Sydney · Tokyo

Acquisitions Editor: Richard Winters
Developmental Editor: Alexandra T. Anderson
Production Editor: Jeff Somers
Manufacturing Manager: Colin J. Warnock
Cover Designer: Mark Lerner
Compositor: Lippincott Williams & Wilkins Desktop Division
Printer: Edwards Brothers

© 2000 by LIPPINCOTT WILLIAMS & WILKINS
530 Walnut Street
Philadelphia, PA 19106 USA
LWW.com

Printed in the USA

Library of Congress Cataloging-in-Publication Data
Spencer, Jeanne M.
   Children's health / Jeanne P. Spencer with Orlando F. Mills.
     p. ; cm.—(The academy collection—quick reference guides for family physicians)
   Includes bibliographical references and index.
   ISBN 0-7817-2052-4 (alk. paper)
   1. Pediatrics. I. Mills, Orlando F. II. Title. III. Series.
   [DNLM: 1. Pediatrics. 2. Child Welfare. WS 100 S745c 2000]
RJ45.S73 2000
618.92—dc21
                                               00-039132

10 9 8 7 6 5 4 3 2 1

CONTENTS

....

ACKNOWLEDGMENTS

I thank my teachers, colleagues, and friends for patience and guidance over the years and for assistance with the writing of this manuscript.

Thanks also to my patients, sons, and foster children for teaching me so much about being a child.

Finally, thanks to my husband, Rob, for his constant encouragement, support, and tolerance.

PREFACE

My goal in the writing of this book was to create a volume to assist the busy family physician with the office care of pediatric patients. Because I work in a rural setting, I have tried to address the particular needs of physicians who may not have access to pediatric subspecialists. Because most children are generally healthy, I have emphasized care of well children of all ages. I have included current immunization recommendations, although I caution the clinician that these change with amazing rapidity.

In writing this book, I have been challenged by the lack of evidence-based information regarding common pediatric problems. Although it is relatively easy to find information on rare metabolic disorders, searching for information on common topics like head lice or growing pains has been difficult. I continue to wonder why information on many problems I see in the office or when precepting residents is not included in pediatric text books, even those on ambulatory pediatrics. It is my hope to fill a portion of this void.

In a similar way, breast-feeding is universally recognized as the preferred method of infant nutrition. Nevertheless, I have found few resources that are useful for primary care physicians seeing breast-feeding patients. I am indebted to authors such as Thomas Hale, Ph.D., and Jack Newman, M.D., who are beginning to publish this information.

I have included a chapter on children in foster care because I have participated in their care as a foster parent and as a physician. Although foster parents make the news only when they are accused of wrongdoing, most foster parents are altruistic and work hard to improve the lives of the children in their care. As physicians, we can work to support foster parents and advocate for the services, especially mental health and educational, that foster children require.

Finally, as family physicians we bring so much to the care of our young patients. We possess skills that our pediatric colleagues often lack, such as the ability to perform pelvic exams. I frequently care for children, parents, and grandparents in the same family, at times during the same visit. This appreciation of the family dynamic enhances the care of the child and makes the interaction more enjoyable. Adolescents are at a pivotal time of life, and we as family physicians have the opportunity to influence the course of the rest of their lives. Of course talking to them can be a challenge, but with a little effort on our part, it is often possible for them to make eye contact with more than their sneakers. As soon as a bond is made, it often carries through to their care as adults, potentially for many years.

Caring for children is fun. A discussion about Teletubbies or smiling at a 4-month-old can be so refreshing in a long day. I hope this book is useful and appreciate your comments.

Jeanne P. Spencer

SERIES INTRODUCTION

Family practice is a unique clinical specialty encompassing a philosophy of care rather than a modality of care provided to a specific segment of the population. This philosophy of providing longitudinal care for persons of all ages in the complete context of their physical, emotional, and social environments was modeled by general practitioners, the parents of our modern specialty. To provide this kind of care, the family physician needs a broad knowledge base, appropriate evaluation tools, effective interventions, and patient education.

The knowledge base needed by a family physician is extraordinarily large. The American Academy of Family Physicians and other organizations provide clinical education to practitioners through conferences and journals. Individual family physicians have written journal articles about specific clinical topics or have tried to cover the broad knowledge base of family medicine in a single volume. The former are helpful, but may cover only a narrow segment of medicine, while the latter may not provide the depth needed to be useful in actual patient care.

The Academy Collection: Quick Reference Guides for Family Physicians is a series of books designed to assist family physicians with the broad knowledge base unique to our specialty. The books in this series have all been written by practicing family physicians who have special interest in the topics, and the chapters have been formatted to provide easy access to information needed at varying stages in the physician-patient encounter. Each volume is unique because each author has personalized the volume and provided a unique family physician perspective.

This series is not meant to be a final reference for the family physician who seeks a comprehensive text. The series also does not cover every topic that may be encountered by the family physician. The series does offer, in a depth deemed appropriate by the authors, the information needed by the physician to handle the majority of patient encounters. The series also provides information to make patient care a combined doctor-patient effort. Specific patient education materials have been included where appropriate. Readers can contact the American Academy of Family Physicians Foundation for other resources.

The topics selected for *The Academy Collection* were chosen based on what family physicians said they needed. The first group of books covers office procedures, conditions of aging, and some of the most challenging diagnoses seen in family practice. Future books in the series will address musculoskeletal problems, environmental medicine, children's health, gastrointestinal problems, and women's health issues.

I welcome your comments. Please contact me at the American Academy of Family Physicians with your suggestions (Rick Sadovsky, MD, Series Editor, *The Academy Collection*, c/o AAFP, 11400 Tomahawk Creek Parkway, Leawood, KS 66211-2672; e-mail: academycollection@aafp.org). This collection is meant to be useful to you and your patients.

Richard Sadovsky, M.D., M.S.
Series Editor

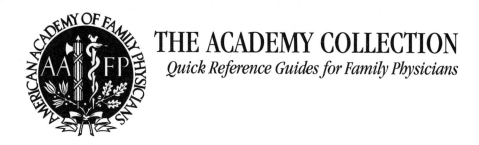

THE ACADEMY COLLECTION
Quick Reference Guides for Family Physicians

Children's Health

CHAPTER 1

. . . .

Newborn

Breastfeeding

Breastfeeding is universally recognized as the optimal method of feeding human infants. The benefits of breastfeeding include a reduction in infectious disease risk, prevention of allergy, and possibly improved intelligence. Breastfeeding mothers have a decreased breast cancer risk, improved child spacing, and quicker return to prepregnancy weight. Since breastfed infants have fewer illnesses, parents lose less time from work. Using 1993 data, breastfeeding a child for 1 year was estimated to save $400 in

TABLE 1.1. Barriers to breastfeeding initiation and continuation

Physician apathy
Physician misinformation and lack of physician education
Inadequate prenatal education
Inadequate postnatal education
Disruptive hospital policies
Cultural bias against breastfeeding
Lack of family support
Early return to work outside the home
Commercial promotion of infant formula

TABLE 1.2. Ten steps to successful breastfeeding: a joint WHO/UNICEF statement (1989)

Every facility providing maternity services and care for newborns should:
1. Have a written breastfeeding policy that is communicated routinely to all health care staff.
2. Train all health care staff in the skills necessary to implement this policy.
3. Inform all pregnant women about the benefits and management of breastfeeding.
4. Help mothers initiate breastfeeding within 30 minutes of birth.
5. Show mothers how to breastfeed and how to maintain lactation even if they are separated from their infants.
6. Give newborns no food or drink other than human milk unless medically indicated.
7. Practice rooming-in: Allow mothers and infants to stay together 24 hours a day.
8. Encourage breastfeeding on demand.
9. Give no artificial teats or pacifiers (also called dummies and soothers) to breastfeeding infants.
10. Foster the establishment of breastfeeding support groups and refer mothers to them on discharge from hospital or clinic.

food costs alone. Despite these unique benefits of breast milk, the United States continues to fall short of the Healthy People 2000 targets of 75% of women initiating breastfeeding and 50% continuing until the child is 5 to 6 months old. Table 1.1 lists barriers to successful breastfeeding initiation and continuation.

To overcome these barriers, physicians need to educate themselves about care of the breastfeeding dyad. We also need to work to implement breastfeeding-friendly hospital policies and to advocate for insurance support of outpatient lactation services. Table 1.2 lists ten steps to successful breastfeeding recommended by the World Health Organization.

GETTING STARTED

The first days of the child's life are often the most difficult time for the breastfeeding dyad. The first step is perfecting the latch-on (Fig. 1.1). The baby should open the

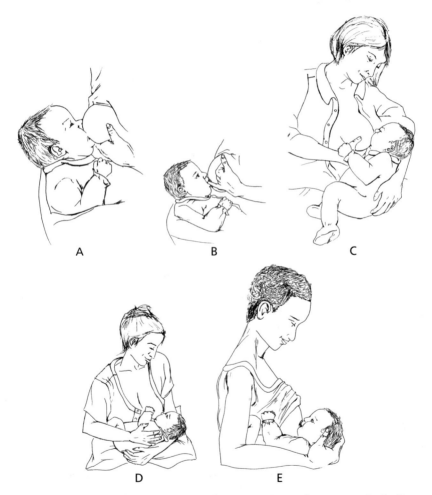

FIGURE 1.1.   A: Latch-on position. **B:** Breaking suction. **C:** Lying-down position. **D:** Cradle position. **E:** Football hold.

mouth wide as in a yawn and be facing directly forward. When removing the baby from the breast, the mother should break the suction with her finger. Varying position (Fig. 1.1) decreases the risk of sore nipples.

In the postpartum period, mothers experience the stress of physical recovery while adapting to the new role of mother. While establishing breastfeeding, mothers should avoid nonessential tasks and elicit the help of support people. Adequate fluid intake and rest are essential. Supplements and pacifiers may hinder the infant's ability to nurse at the breast and so should be avoided until breastfeeding is well established.

GETTING ENOUGH

In the early weeks of breastfeeding, health care providers and mothers need to monitor adequacy of caloric intake (Table 1.3).

Mothers should nurse when early hunger cues, such as increased alertness or activity, mouthing or rooting, are seen, typically eight to 12 times daily. Since the first few days at home are a pivotal time for the nursing dyad, they should be evaluated in the first 2 to 4 days after discharge. This may be done either in the office or at home, depending on the mother's and provider's circumstances. In many cases a home visit by a provider experienced in lactation is ideal.

ENGORGEMENT

Engorgement may occur when the milk first comes in, usually days 3 to 6, or it may occur at any time when the frequency of breastfeeding is abruptly reduced. In engorgement the breasts become enlarged, firm, and tender. In the newborn period, breastfeeding frequently and well decreases the risk of painful engorgement. If engorgement flattens the nipple, the baby may have difficulty latching on. Expressing some milk either manually or with a pump softens the nipple, facilitates latch-on, and allows the child to remove the milk from the breast. Between feedings, cold compresses and acetaminophen may give symptomatic relief. Cabbage leaves may also help. To use them, raw, green cabbage leaves are crushed with a rolling pin, and a hole is cut out for the nipple. The leaves are then applied to the breasts and worn in the bra twice daily for 20 minutes. Typically, the engorgement decreases after two or three applications. Women with this degree of difficulty with nursing are at high risk of discontinuation and need close follow-up.

SORE NIPPLES

Sore nipples are one of the most common reasons for discontinuing nursing, and any pain beyond brief discomfort at the initiation of nursing is not normal. In the early

TABLE 1.3.   Signs of successful breastfeeding

Audible swallowing
Eight to 10 feedings daily
Colorless, dilute urine six to eight times daily (once the milk comes in)
Three to five yellow, seedy stools daily (once the milk comes in)
Weight gain by 4 or 5 days of age
Back to birth weight by 2 weeks of age

T ABLE 1.4.   Treatment of candidal infections

Infant

Nystatin suspension (Mycostatin)	2 mL, apply to the mouth	4 times daily × 14 days
Gentian violet 0.5% to 1%*	0.1 mL, apply to the mouth	daily × 4 days
Fluconazole (Diflucan)†	6 mg/kg, first day, then 3 mg/kg	daily × 2 weeks

Mother

Nystatin ointment (Mycolog II)	Apply to the nipple/areola	after each feeding × 14 days
Clotrimazole cream (Lotrimin)	Apply to the nipple/areola	after each feeding × 14 days
Gentian violet, 0.5% to 1%*	0.1 mL, apply to the mouth	daily × 4 days
Fluconazole†	200 mg, first dose, then 100 mg	daily × 2 weeks

*To use gentian violet have the infant suck on a cotton swab dipped in the gentian violet. If the entire mouth is not covered, the mouth can be painted with an additional swab. The child should then nurse. If both nipples are not covered at the end of the feeding, the nipple can be painted directly. Gentian violet can be used simultaneously with other treatments. Bedtime treatment with the baby dressed in only a diaper can reduce staining.

†Not FDA approved.

days, sore nipples are most often due to poor latch-on. Often, varying the position and reemphasizing proper technique alleviate the problem (see earlier).

Breast pads may exacerbate sore nipples because they keep the nipples moist. Nipples should be exposed to the open air as much as possible. Applying expressed breast milk or purified lanolin (Lansinoh) to the nipple may help. If the problem persists and the latch is correct, a combination of an antistaphylococcal antibiotic, antifungal, and antiinflammatory cream (Mycolog II and bactroban) applied sparingly after feedings may help.

Rhythmic motions of the tongue are needed to express milk from the nipple. Any impediment to this motion such as that due to a short frenulum, prematurity, or neurologic abnormalities may result in poor let-down and sore nipples. Observation of a feeding, including latch and suck, is essential in the evaluation of sore nipples. Clipping of a short frenulum has been shown to improve nursing.

Candidal infections of the nipple are also common. Often mothers with such infections complain of intense burning or stabbing pain with nursing. This may occur immediately post partum or months into nursing. Candidal infection is particularly common when the infant has diaper dermatitis or the mother has vaginal candidiasis. Frequently the nipple appears normal, although it may have mild to severe erythema, scaling, cracks, or fissures. Fungal culture of the skin or milk is not helpful. Simultaneous treatment of the mother and infant is essential to avoid recurrent infection. Usually, the child and mother can be treated topically, but systemic treatment may be needed in more severe or recalcitrant cases (Table 1.4). The application of a moderate-strength steroid cream such as 0.1% triamcinolone to the nipple may speed resolution of the symptoms. Persistent yeast in the home environment may be a source of reinfection. In these cases clothing, items in contact with the baby's mouth, and bed linens should be cleaned in boiling or hot water.

BLOCKED MILK DUCTS

Blocked ducts present as tender, firm, reddened, wedge-shaped areas of the breast. Fever and malaise are not seen. Treatment is frequent breastfeeding, with the baby's chin placed toward the area of the blockage. Milk expression, heat, and massage may

T ABLE 1.5.   Antibiotics for the treatment of mastitis

Cephalexin (Keflex)	500 mg four times daily
Dicloxacillin	250 mg four times daily
Clindamycin (Cleocin)	500 mg four times daily

help. Acetaminophen may relieve the pain. A blocked duct may progress to mastitis if not treated; any presumed blocked duct lasting more than 48 hours should be examined to confirm the diagnosis.

MASTITIS

Mastitis may clinically resemble a blocked duct. The breast is firm, tender, and erythematous in a wedge-shaped area. The presence of fever, malaise, and myalgias in the mother usually distinguishes this from a blocked duct. *Staphylococcus aureus* is the usual infecting organism, and antibiotic treatment is recommended for at least 10 to 14 days (Table 1.5).

The infant should continue nursing, starting on the uninfected side to decrease the mother's discomfort. Since the infecting organism is usually already present in the flora of the infant's mouth, there is little risk of infecting the infant. Manual milk expression or gentle pumping may be possible if the breast is too sore when nursing. Abrupt cessation of nursing may result in increased pain and progression to abscess. Supportive treatment with acetaminophen and bedrest are recommended.

BREAST ABSCESS

The mother presents with a very tender, firm mass in the breast, often following untreated mastitis or a blocked duct. Needle aspiration yields purulent material, or the abscess may be seen on ultrasound. Treatment is incision and drainage of the abscess accompanied by oral antibiotics, as for mastitis. Office incision and drainage under local anesthesia is similar to that for abscesses in the nonlactating breast. The incision is best placed perpendicular to the areola (parallel to the milk ducts) and as far away from the nipple as possible to facilitate further nursing.

RETURN TO WORK

Many nursing mothers continue nursing after they return to work. Some mothers choose to work part time; others either pump or nurse their children during breaks. Most mothers save the expressed milk for use when they are away. If the mother chooses not to pump while away from the child and if the timing of nursing is consistent, the breasts produce more milk at the times of day the mother usually nurses. This is more effective if the mother works consistent shifts. Many infants nurse more frequently when the mother is available and less when the mother is away. For many mothers, continued nursing strengthens their bond to their child and may diminish guilt feelings about being away for work. Many mothers continue to nurse in the mornings and at night for prolonged periods of time.

BREAST PUMPS

The three main types of breast pumps are manual, minielectric, and larger electric pumps. Dual pumping facilitates the let-down reflex and is best for prolonged pumping. Manual pumps are inexpensive, but the muscles in the hands tire quickly. Foot pumps can be very effective. Minielectric pumps are convenient in size and may be battery operated. Rental, double electric pumps are best if pumping is planned for a prolonged period, such as return to work or to maintain milk production during prolonged separation from the child or if the child has special needs, such as those of the premature infant. Additional information on breast pumps may be obtained from the vendors listed below. Some family practices choose to become pump rental stations to facilitate access to breast pumps. Breast milk may be stored for 6 hours at room temperature, 2 days in the refrigerator, 3 months in a freezer with a door separate from the refrigerator, and 6 months in a deep freeze. Sterile disposable plastic bottle liners are ideal for freezing breast milk.

MATERNAL ILLNESS

Many questions about breastfeeding arise when the mother becomes ill herself. Table 1.6 lists maternal infectious diseases and breastfeeding recommendations. Mothers may continue to nurse with common bacterial and viral illnesses, such as upper respiratory infections.

MEDICATIONS

Use of medications is one of the most common reasons women are told to stop breastfeeding. Unfortunately, many of these recommendations are unfounded. Table 1.7 lists medications that are safe in the nursing mother. For medications not listed here, the Hale text is an excellent, quick resource; in addition, the Lactation Study Center provides phone consultation. When any medication is used, Table 1.8 lists helpful pointers.

T ABLE 1.6.   Breastfeeding with maternal infectious diseases

Disease	Recommendation
Tuberculosis	Separate mother and baby until maternal sputum is negative, usually 2 weeks
HIV	Avoid breastfeeding in developed countries
Hepatitis A	Breastfeeding permitted, give infant gamma globulin if infection is within 2 weeks of birth
Hepatitis B	Breastfeeding may begin once infant receives hepatitis B immune globulin
Hepatitis C	Breastfeeding permitted
Herpes simplex	Avoid breastfeeding if the lesions are on the breast
	If lesions are elsewhere, they should be covered and the mother should wash her hands before holding the baby
Varicella zoster	If infection is within 6 days of birth and child has no lesions, isolate mother and baby, give infant varicella immune globulin.
	May resume nursing when mother is noninfectious.

Adapted from Lawrence RA. *A review of the medical benefits and contraindications to breastfeeding in the United States.* Arlington, VA: National Center for Education in Maternal and Child Health, 1997.

T ABLE 1.7. Medication safe to use in normal doses for mothers nursing healthy full-term infants

Acetaminophen
Antacids
Carbamazepine (Tegretol)
Cephalosporins
Cetirizine (Zyrtec)
Clindamycin (Cleocin)
Clotrimazole (Lotrimin)
Codeine
Decongestant nasal sprays
Digoxin (Lanoxin)
Erythromycin
Fluconazole
Heparin
Ibuprofen (Motrin)
Inhalers—bronchodilators, steroid
Insulin
Laxatives—bulk-forming, stool softeners
Lidocaine (Xylocaine)
Penicillins
Prednisone
Propranolol (Inderal)
Vaccines
Warfarin (Coumadin)

Adapted from American Academy of Pediatrics Committee on Drugs. The transfer of drugs and other chemicals into human milk. *Pediatrics* 1994;93:137; and Hale, TW. *Medications and mother's milk,* 7th ed. Amarillo, TX: Pharmasoft Medical Publishing, 1998.

T ABLE 1.8. Decreasing the risk of medications used by nursing mothers

1. Use medication only when needed
2. If the medication is safe to prescribe directly to an infant the age of the nursing child, it is safe in the breastmilk
3. If a medication cannot be absorbed orally, it cannot be absorbed from the breastmilk
4. Dose medications after nursing
5. Dose once-daily medications before the child's longest sleep period
6. Choose medications with the shortest half-life
7. Choose medications with the lowest oral bioavailability

WEANING

The decision to wean is an individualized one. The American Academy of Pediatrics recommends that breastfeeding be continued for 1 year and as long after that as desired by the infant and mother. Iron-fortified foods should be gradually introduced in the second half of the first year. Some infants wean themselves by gradually replacing breastfeeding with solids. If the mother desires to wean, gradually eliminating breastfeedings allows for a slow reduction in milk supply and so minimizes the risk of engorgement.

REFERRAL

Family physicians vary widely in interest and expertise in assisting the breastfeeding mother. Lactation consultants specialize in the management of breastfeeding problems, including breastfeeding technique, alternative feeding methods, and the use of breast pumps. Many are credentialed by the International Board of Certified Lactation Consultants (IBCLC), and may be nurses, experienced lay people, dietitians, and physicians. They may be found through their professional organization (see later). In some areas breastfeeding centers are also available.

REFERENCES

American Academy of Pediatrics Committee on Drugs. The transfer of drugs and other chemicals into human milk. *Pediatrics* 1994;93:137.

American Academy of Pediatrics Work Group on Breastfeeding. Breastfeeding and the use of human milk. *Pediatrics* 1997;100:1035.

Hale, TW. *Medications and mothers' milk,* 7th ed. Amarillo, TX: Pharmasoft Medical Publishing, 1998.

Lawrence RA. *A review of the medical benefits and contraindications to breastfeeding in the United States.* (Maternal and Child Health Technical Information Bulletin). Arlington, VA: National Center for Education in Maternal and Child Health, 1997.

Lawrence RA. *Breastfeeding: a guide for the medical profession*, 4th ed. St Louis: Mosby, 1994.

Melnikow J, Bedinghouse JM. Management of common breast feeding problems. *J Fam Pract* 1994;39:56.

Mohrbacher N, Stock J. *The breastfeeding answer book.* Schaumburg, IL: La Leche League International, 1997.

Neifert M. Early assessment of the breastfeeding infant. *Contemp Pediatr* October 1996;13(10)142.

Newman J. Sore breasts: diagnosis and treatment. *Can J Pediatr* 1996;7:472.

Newman J. Treating sore nipples. *Can J Pediatr* 1996;7:436.

Powers NG, Slusser W,. Breastfeeding update 2: clinical lactation management. *Pediatr Rev* 1997;18:147.

Slusser W, Powers NG. Breastfeeding update 1: immunology, nutrition, and advocacy. *Pediatr Rev* 1997;18:111.

Spencer JP. Practical nutrition for the healthy term infant. *Am Fam Physician* 1996;54:138.

Breast Pump Vendors

Hollister/Ameda/Egnell. 800-624-4060. www.hollister.com

Medela, Inc. 800-435-8316. www.medela.com

White River Concepts. 800-824-6351. www.whiteriver.com

Patient Education

La Leche League International, Inc. *The womanly art of breastfeeding,* 6th ed. Schaumberg, IL: La Leche League International, 1997.

Renfrew M, Fisher C, Arms S. Bestfeeding: getting breastfeeding right for you. Berkeley, CA: Celestial Arts, 1990.

Tamaro, Janet. *So that's what they're for!: breastfeeding basics,* 2nd ed. Holbrook, MA: Adams Media Corporation, 1998.

Lactation Consultant Location

International Lactation Consultant Association. 312-541-1710.

Professional Textbooks

Briggs GG, Freeman RY, Yaffe SJ. *Drugs in pregnancy and lactation,* 5th ed. Baltimore: Williams & Wilkins, 1998. (Thorough review of medications used in lactation.)

Hale TW. *Medications and mothers' milk,* 7th ed. Amarillo, TX: Pharmasoft Medical Publishing, 1998. (Inexpensive, thorough, practical review of medications. To order call 800-378-1317.)

Lawrence RA. *Breastfeeding: a guide for the medical profession,* 4th ed. St Louis, MO: Mosby, 1994. (Thorough review of the research on breastfeeding.)

Mohrbacher N, Stock J. *The breastfeeding answer book.* Schaumberg, IL: La Leche League International, 1997. (Very practical review. Great for office staff.)

Professional Information

Lactation Study Center, University of Rochester. 716-275-0088 (8 A.M. to 5 P.M. EST). (Information on lactation or medications in lactation; usually answer questions immediately. Comprehensive breastfeeding database.)

Internet

Dr. Hale's Breastfeeding Pharmacology page. neonatal.ttuhsc.edu/lact/

La Leche League. www.lalecheleague.org. Bookstore, patient education.

LACTNET. www.telcomplus.net/kga/LACTNET.HTM. Email discussion list for professionals.

Continuing Medical Education

La Leche League. 800-LA-LECHE. www.lalecheleague.org. Host local professional education conferences and the Annual Seminar for Physicians cosponsored by the American Academy of Family Physicians (AAFP).

Lactation Education Resources. 301-986-5547. www.leron-line.com/index.htm. (Sponsors week-long lactation education courses.)

Formula Feeding

FORMULA SELECTION

The lay press advises parents to contact their physician about the formula that is best suited for their child. In reality, this decision is usually quite arbitrary, and after breast milk, a cow's milk–based formula is usually the first choice for a healthy, term infant. Iron-fortified formulas are best, because low-iron formulas have not been shown to be better tolerated by infants and are associated with iron deficiency. If parents insist on low-iron formula, they should periodically be encouraged to retry iron-fortified formula, and hemoglobin levels should be monitored, usually at 6 to 9 months. Soy formula is free of cow's milk protein and lactose. Soy formulas have no advantage over cow's milk–based formulas for supplementation in the breastfed infant, prevention of colic, prevention of atopic disease, or amelioration of gastroenteritis unless lactose intolerance is documented. Soy formulas are compatible with a vegetarian diet and do meet the full-term child's nutritional needs. Protein hydrolysate formulas contain hydrolyzed protein, which is not antigenic. Because of their high cost, poor taste, and high osmolality, their use should be restricted to medically necessary situations, such as intolerance to soy and cow's milk–based formula, or malabsorption syndromes. Table 1.9 lists the names and types of various formulas. Specialized formulas are available for use in premature infants and infants with inborn errors of metabolism.

Formulas are sold as ready-to-feed formula, liquid concentrate, and powder, in order of decreasing cost. Ready-to-feed formula is convenient to prepare and is especially useful for travel. Liquid concentrate must be diluted 1:1 with water and is supplied by the Women, Infants, and Children Program (WIC) to their clients. Powdered formula must be diluted with 2 ounces of water per scoop. Parents must measure the diluting water accurately, especially for newborns, and the powder must be dissolved completely. The need for sterilizing bottles, nipples, and water used in bottle preparation is debated. Formula manufacturers recommend sterilization. Others argue that if bottles are used immediately after preparation, sterilization is unnecessary. Unsanitized water, such as well water, should be boiled for 1 minute. Before use, cold tapwater should be allowed to run for approximately 2 minutes to clear the pipes of contaminants such as lead.

Bottle-fed infants are more likely to adhere to a schedule than breastfed infants. Newborns generally have six to eight feedings daily, and estimated consumption is one-half of their weight (pounds) of formula (ounces). Formula may be consumed either warm or cold. Warming the bottle in warm water is safest. Bottles should not be microwaved, as overheated areas develop quickly.

FORMULA INTOLERANCE

Formula intolerance is difficult to diagnose. Some infants have allergic reactions to cow's milk proteins and are at risk of having similar allergic reactions to soy proteins,

T ABLE 1.9. Infant formulas

Cow's Milk Based	Soy	Protein Hydrolysate
Enfamil with Iron	Isomil with Iron	Nutramagen
Similac with Iron	Prosobee with Iron	Alimentum

because both are foreign proteins. In this case an elemental formula should be used. Other infants may be lactose intolerant and thus would do well with a soy formula. Other conditions, such as colic, may be mistakenly blamed on formula intolerance. These infants may improve with formula substitution even within the same type. Constipation is common in the formula-fed infant and may improve with a change of formula brand or type.

REFERENCES

Committee on Nutrition. American Academy of Pediatrics. *Pediatric nutrition handbook.* Elk Grove, IL: American Academy of Pediatrics, 1998.

Committee on Nutrition. American Academy of Pediatrics. Soy Protein-based formulas: recommendations for use in infant feeding. *Pediatrics* 1998;101:148.

Spencer, JP. Practical nutrition for the healthy term infant. *Am Fam Physician* 1996;54:138. (Includes patient education handout.)

Jaundice

CHIEF COMPLAINT

"My newborn child is yellow."

HISTORY OF THE PRESENT ILLNESS

With the acceleration of hospital discharge, evaluation of the jaundiced newborn has moved to the outpatient setting. This evaluation begins with assessment of the general well-being of the child. As any severe illness in the newborn may present as jaundice, careful attention must be paid to signs of sepsis, such as fever, temperature instability, apnea, behavioral changes, persistent vomiting, or persistent feeding difficulties. In the breastfeeding child, the detailed feeding history should include frequency, duration, maternal discomfort, and presence of rhythmic sucking and swallowing during feeds, because inadequate breastfeeding is a common cause of hyperbilirubinemia. The number of wet and soiled diapers and presence of urate crystals or dark discoloration of the urine (conjugated hyperbilirubinemia) and characteristics of the bowel movement should be assessed.

FAMILY HISTORY

Specific inquiry should be made into a family history of hemolytic anemia, severe jaundice, and ethnicity or geographic origin associated with hemolytic anemia.

PHYSICAL EXAMINATION

The examination should focus on signs of underlying disease that may be causing the jaundice. In particular, the temperature, respiratory rate, and weight should be noted. Additionally, the alertness and muscle tone of the child, lung sounds and presence of heart murmurs, hepatomegaly, and splenomegaly are particularly important. Rashes should be noted. The level of bilirubin can be assessed by applying pressure to the skin and noting the level of yellow coloration (Table 1.10).

T ABLE   1.10.   Approximate bilirubin levels for various levels of anatomic
progression

Bilirubin concentration

Face	~5 mg/dL
Mid-abdomen	~15 mg/dL
Soles	~20 mg/dL

LABORATORY EVALUATION

A total serum bilirubin level should be measured in all infants with moderate jaundice
or jaundice that reaches the level of the midabdomen. Other evaluation is guided by
Fig. 1.2.

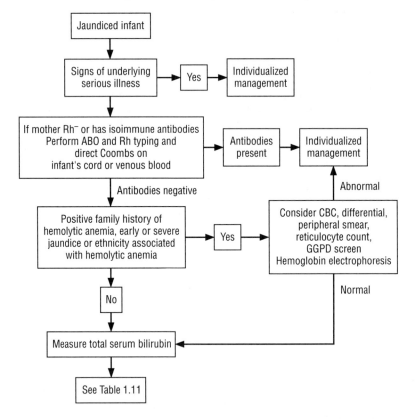

FIGURE 1.2.   Jaundice management for healthy newborn past the age of 37 weeks.

DIFFERENTIAL DIAGNOSIS

The differential diagnosis of the jaundiced infant is quite broad. As even the healthy newborn's immature liver may be unable to meet the demands of bilirubin metabolism (physiologic jaundice), any condition that stresses the newborn, including infection and hypoxia, may result in jaundice. Bilirubin is recycled through the enterohepatic circulation, so any condition that slows transport through the gut can lead to increased bilirubin recycling and hyperbilirubinemia. Hemolysis either due to a hematologic condition or to the breakdown of blood, such as in a hematoma, results in metabolism of excess bilirubin and may lead to jaundice. Breastfeeding jaundice is the direct result of inadequate nutritional support and is analogous to adult starvation jaundice. It occurs in the first week of life and is caused by inadequate breastfeeding, not by any factor intrinsic to breast milk. Breast milk jaundice typically occurs in the second or third weeks of life and may continue for up to 3 months. This is seen in infants who are nursing and gaining well. This condition is thought to be caused by an as yet undiscovered factor in breast milk. It is not associated with kernicterus.

Kernicterus results from the deposition of unconjugated bilirubin in the brainstem. Its early manifestations include lethargy, changes in muscle tone, seizures, and opisthotonus. Choreoathetoid cerebral palsy, hearing loss, and upward gaze palsy are seen later in the course of the disease.

MANAGEMENT

Management of the jaundiced infant has long been controversial. In full-term infants most studies have failed to document an association between the bilirubin level and future intelligence or neurologic outcome. In 1994 the American Academy of Pediatrics published a Practice Parameter on the Management of Hyperbilirubinemia in the Healthy Term Infant (Table 1.11) based mostly on retrospective epidemiologic

T ABLE 1.11. Management of hyperbilirubinemia in the healthy term and near-term newborn

	TSB Level [mg/dL (μmol/L)]			
Age (h)	Consider Phototherapy*	Phototherapy	Exchange Transfusion if Intensive Phototherapy Fails†	Exchange Transfusion and Intensive Phototherapy
≤24‡	—	—	—	—
25–48	≥12 (205)	≥15 (260)	≥20 (340)	≥25 (430)
49–72	≥15 (260)	≥18 (310)	≥25 (430)	≥30 (510)
>72	≥17 (290)	≥20 (340)	≥25 (430)	≥30 (510)

Abbreviation: TSB, total serum bilirubin.

*Phototherapy at these TSB levels is a clinical option, meaning that the intervention is available and may be used on the basis of individual clinical judgment.

†Intensive phototherapy should produce a decline of TSB of 1 to 2 mg/dL within 4–6 hours and the TSB level should continue to fall and remain below the threshold level for exchange transfusion. If this does not occur, it is considered a failure of phototherapy.

‡Term infants who are clinically jaundiced at ≤24 hours old are not considered healthy and require further evaluation.

Reprinted with permission from Management of hyperbilirubinemia in the Healthy Term Newborn. *Practice Guideline.* 1994; Elk Grove Village, Illinois: American Academy of Pediatrics.

data, since no large-scale clinical trial has been done. Madlon-Kay, in a recent study of family physicians, found that their practice patterns were similar but not identical to the guidelines. Interestingly, many family physicians recommended increased sunlight exposure for jaundiced infants; unfortunately, this has not been studied since 1958.

In breastfed infants, management of feeding issues is especially important. Optimal breastfeeding from the start would eliminate much of the jaundice in these infants. Breastfeeding jaundice is managed primarily by enhancing breastfeeding technique and milk supply. Although formula supplementation may be effective and easily implemented, the mother and child are at risk of discontinuation of breastfeeding. When the infant is undernourished and the breastfeeding is inadequate, formula supplementation in addition to improved breastfeeding may be needed. Pumping the breasts after feedings often helps to stimulate the milk supply.

In breast milk jaundice, babies appear healthy and gain weight well. The bilirubin peaks at 2 to 3 weeks and may remain elevated for 3 months. If the bilirubin remains below 20 mg/dL, no intervention is needed. For higher levels, 24 hours of formula supplementation with pumping and storage of the breast milk for later use may be effective. Phototherapy, often at home, may also be effective. Some argue that since breast milk jaundice has never been shown to be harmful to the infant, no intervention is needed, regardless of the bilirubin level.

REFERRAL

Management of infants of less than 37 weeks gestation, infants with jaundice in the first 24 hours of life, or infants who appear ill often requires specialist evaluation. Referral to a lactation consultant may be quite beneficial in breastfeeding jaundice. Specialist referral may also be needed for hematologic abnormalities or if the child does not respond to standard management.

REFERENCES

Gartner LM. Neonatal jaundice. *Pediatr Rev* 1994;15:422.

Madlon-Kay DJ. Evaluation and management of newborn jaundice by Midwest family physicians. *J Fam Pract* 1998;47:461.

Neifert M. Early assessment of the breastfeeding infant. *Contemp Pediatr* October 1996;13(10)142.

Provisional Committee for Quality Improvement and Subcommittee on Hyperbilirubinemia. Practice parameter on the management of hyperbilirubinemia in the healthy term newborn. *Pediatrics* 1994;94:558.

CHAPTER 2

··

Well-Child Visits

Well-child visits are an integral part of pediatric care. Although parents may view these visits as "shot visits," much of their benefit comes from the assessment of the child and the guidance given to the parents. Haber has shown that early detection of developmental delay has resulted in improved outcomes for children. Each visit should cover five main areas:

Interval history/parental concerns

Physical assessment

Developmental assessment

Anticipatory guidance

Health maintenance

The specifics of these areas for the various ages will be reviewed later. As each child and family situation is unique, the assessment and guidance should be individualized. Similarly, the frequency of the visits should be adjusted to suit the needs of the particular child and family setting. The following visits are the ages that well-child examinations are frequently performed in family practice offices. The U.S. Preventive Services Task Force report finds data regarding the optimum frequency of these visits to be lacking. The American Academy of Pediatrics recommends more frequent visits. More frequent visits may be appropriate in the following situations:

Chronically ill child

Behavioral problems

Foster or adoptive child

Increased parental anxiety

Parental mental or physical illness

Socially or economically disadvantaged child

Well-child care can often be incorporated into visits for an acute problem. This is particularly necessary for adolescents, who are less likely to present for well-child care. Finally, no physician can cover the pertinent parenting information for a particular age in a single office visit, and if it were possible, no parent could retain it. Handouts, videos, parenting texts, parenting classes, community programs, or in-home services (in highest-risk situations) can supplement office visits.

Growth charts are essential throughout the childhood years. Remember to praise the parents for their efforts.

REFERENCES

American Academy of Pediatrics, Committee on Infectious Diseases. Update on tuberculosis skin testing of children. *Pediatrics* 1996;97:282.

Guidelines for health supervision III. Elk Grove Village, Illinois: American Academy of Pediatrics, 1997.

Well child care reference guide, 7th ed. Lexington, Kentucky: American Board of Family Practice, 1998.

Haber JS. Early diagnosis and referral of children with developmental disabilities. *Am Fam Physician* 1991;43:132.

U.S. Preventive Services Task Force. *Guide to clinical preventive services,* 2nd ed. Baltimore: Williams & Wilkins, 1996.

U.S. Public Health Service. *Put prevention into practice: clinician's handbook of preventive services,* 2nd ed. McLean, VA: International Medical Publishing, 1998.

Unti SM. The critical first year of life. *Pediatr Clin North Am* 1994;41:859.

Patient Resources/Education

American Academy of Family Physicians (AAFP). Family health and medical guide. Nashville, Tennessee: Word Publishing, 1996.

American Academy of Pediatrics. *Caring for your baby and young child: birth to age 5.* New York: Bantam Doubleday Dell, 1998.

American Academy of Pediatrics guide to your child's symptoms. New York: Villard Books, 1999.

Eisenberg A, Murkoff H, Hathaway S. *What to expect the first year.* New York: Workman, 1996.

Schmidt B. *Your child's health.* New York: Bantam, 1991.

First Office Visit

Recommendations for the timing of the first office visit vary. Traditionally, this visit has been at 2 weeks of age, yet if the child was born at home, was discharged at less than 48 hours, or is breast feeding, this visit should be at age 2 to 7 days. Visits by home health or a lactation consultant may supplement the office visits, especially if the mother cannot travel. Parents of newborns are frequently exhausted and may be unable to absorb information fully. Handouts can supplement verbal advice.

HISTORY

Ask the parents how the child is doing. How is the child feeding? Is he spitting up? Does the breast or bottle feeding seem successful? (See also Chapter 1.) Does the child seem satisfied? Any fever? How frequently is the child wetting and soiling diapers. What is the appearance of the stool? (Expect a yellow, seedy appearance of the stool of the breastfed child.) Are there any concerns about the umbilical cord or its care? How is the child sleeping? Where—on the stomach or back? How frequently does the child awaken at night? How is his or her temperament? Is this child different from previous children (if applicable)? How are the parents coping? Is anyone helping them? How are other family members reacting?

How was the pregnancy? See Table 2.1 for pertinent prenatal history. Parents vary greatly in their ability to recount the prenatal and neonatal history. Ideally, hospital records are available during the office visit. Was the child in the "regular nursery," discharged with mom, given any immunizations or medications? Was the child's hearing screened? What concerns do the parents have?

TABLE 2.1. Prenatal history

Maternal age
Maternal medications
Maternal substance use, including alcohol, cocaine, tobacco
Maternal illness
Maternal infections, including gonorrhea, chlamydia, group B strep, herpes, HIV, syphilis
X-ray exposure
Exposure to teratogens
Concerns on ultrasound
Maternal history of depression
Intrapartum course, including infections, complications, route of delivery
Gestational age or "due date"

FAMILY HISTORY

Are there diseases that run in the family? Was any special genetic screening done during the pregnancy?

SOCIAL HISTORY

Sensitively ask if the pregnancy was planned or desired. Who lives in the home? Who is home to care for the child? What is the long-term child care plan? Is there substance abuse or domestic violence in the home?

PHYSICAL EXAMINATION

Begin the examination by asking the parents if there are any areas of particular concern. At this age the child will usually stay still on the examination table, with the examiner and parent safeguarding him from falls. Check the eyes for red reflex whenever they are open. Check the heart and femoral pulses when the child is quiet. In general, begin with the least invasive aspects of the examination and progress to the more invasive (ears). At this visit the weight is one of the most key elements. The child should be back to birth weight by 10 to 14 days of age.

On the examination, pay particular attention to:

Parent/child interaction—do the parents seem comfortable handling the child?

Weight, length, head circumference

Skin—jaundice, pigmented nevi, rashes, mongoloid spots

Skull—molding, cephalhematoma

Red reflex

Clavicles—evidence of fracture

Neck—torticollis

Chest—breast

Heart—murmur

Abdominal masses, umbilical cord

Hips—dislocatability

Femoral pulses

Genitalia—testes, circumcision, hydrocele

Movement of four limbs

Feet—clubfoot, metatarsus adductus

Neuromotor development

DEVELOPMENT

The 2-week-old should be able to:

Raise head slightly from prone position

Blink to bright light

Focus and follow with eyes

Respond to sounds

ANTICIPATORY GUIDANCE

Many parents have a number of questions at this visit; often they come in with a list. If first-time parents have no questions, this may be a cause for concern. Some are too fatigued to absorb information. Most benefit from a good parent's guide. *Your Child's Health* by Barton Schmitt and *What to Expect the First Year* by Arlene Eisenberg are excellent.

Any illness in the first month of life can be life-threatening. Table 2.2 lists reasons to urgently call the physician. Parents should keep emergency numbers, including the physician, poison control, and emergency medical services (911) near the phone. Discuss night-time office coverage for the practice. Parents should also know which emergency room is best, including proximity and insurance coverage.

To avoid excessive fatigue, parents need to sleep when the child sleeps.

Postpartum blues and depression are common, especially in women who have histories of depression. Many women feel embarrassed about reporting symptoms, espe-

TABLE 2.2.   Reasons to call the physician urgently in the first month

Fever greater than 100ºF
Yellow sclera or skin
Refusal to feed
Unusual irritability
Persistent vomiting
Diarrhea
Somnolence
Breathing difficulty
Does not look well

cially when they have a perfect, desired child. Treatment with counseling or antidepressants can be dramatically effective.

Other anticipatory guidance includes the following:

Don't shake the child; if the child is overly frustrating, put the child in the crib and scream yourself.

Give no solids until the age of 4 months.

Place the baby on his back for sleeping.

Vary the child's head position while she is sleeping on her back.

Remember that touching or washing the fontanelle will not cause harm.

The child should ride in the back seat of the car—never in the front with an operational airbag.

In the car the child should always ride in a backward-facing, approved, infant safety seat.

The infant safety seat needs to be properly belted in the car.

Keep the baby out of direct sunlight.

Sneezing and hiccups are normal.

Breast enlargement and vaginal discharge (even bloody) of the newborn are normal and will resolve.

Take the child's rectal temperature if she seems warm or ill.

Newborns should not be left alone with pets or young siblings.

Temperatures taken with pacifier thermometers, temperature strips, or tympanic thermometers are not generally accurate (Table 2.3).

Table 2.4 lists other anticipatory guidance for this age.

Many parents will need to obtain day care outside the home. If day care is needed for the first months of life, this should ideally be selected before the child is born. Parents should contact other parents of children attending the day care to determine if they are satisfied. Parents should make unannounced visits to inspect the facility. Selecting a day care facility may be one of the most important decisions a parent may make for the young child. Quality can greatly affect the child's experience, and the least expensive facility may not be adequate. Table 2.5 lists other questions for day care providers.

HEALTH MAINTENANCE

If the hepatitis B immunization was not given in the hospital, the thimerosal-free vaccine is given at this visit. Vaccine information sheets may be given in preparation for future immunizations.

COMMON MEDICAL PROBLEMS

Most infants by far are healthy, but early identification of the ill child is critical to prevent rapid deterioration. Many prescription medications are contradicted in the

TABLE 2.3. Taking the child's temperature

1. **Rectal temperature**—most accurate, best in the newborn period, difficult in the squirmy toddler
   a. Shake the glass thermometer so the mercury is below 98ºF or use an electronic one
   b. Lubricate the end of the thermometer with petroleum jelly
   c. Lay the child in your lap
   d. Insert but do not force the thermometer 1 inch
   e. Press the buttocks together
   f. After 2 minutes or when the electronic thermometer beeps, remove the thermometer and write down the temperature
2. **Axillary temperature**—much less accurate; may be only possible method in toddlers
   a. Place the thermometer in the axilla
   b. Hold the elbow against the chest
   c. After 5 minutes or when the electronic thermometer beeps, remove the thermometer and record the temperature
   d. As an approximation, the axillary temperature is 3ºF less than the rectal temperature
3. **Oral temperature**—best way to take temperature in a child greater than 5 years of age
   a. Avoid hot or cold foods for 10–30 minutes before taking the temperature
   b. Place the thermometer under one side of the tongue
   c. Have the child keep the thermometer in place with the lips and fingers (not teeth)
   d. After 3 minutes or when the thermometer beeps, record the temperature
   e. The oral temperature is generally 1ºF less than the rectal temperature

Note: Temperatures taken with pacifier thermometers, temperature strips, or tympanic thermometers are not generally accurate.

neonate because of the immature liver and the risk of the medications displacing bilirubin from albumin, which increases the risk of bilirubin toxicity.

Assessment of the child's growth is one of the most important aspects of the first office visit. The office weight should be compared with the birth weight, and at 10 to 14 days the child should be at least back to birth weight. If the weight is not as expected, a detailed dietary history should be taken, including how frequently the child is being nursed or receiving the bottle. In the formula-fed child, exact amounts of formula consumed should be assessed. Ideally, the breastfed child should be observed nursing to assess latch-on, let-down, and swallowing. If possible, consultation with a lactation consultant can be very valuable. The history should include frequency and amount of spitting up, and daily number of wet and soiled diapers. A careful physical examination should be done to exclude signs of infection. The parent's interaction with the child should be assessed. Table 2.6 lists the most common causes of failure to thrive in this age group.

If a dietary cause is likely, the child's feedings may be improved, and the child can be weighed every 2 to 3 days on the same scale. If a psychosocial cause is suspected, an evaluation by a home nurse can be invaluable. If the child does not improve or worsens, hospital admission and laboratory evaluation are indicated. The exact laboratory evaluation should be directed by the history and physical, but usually includes a complete blood count, electrolytes, and urinalysis.

TABLE **2.4.** Anticipatory guidance: common newborn problems (2-week visit)

Condition	Treatment	Comments
Umbilical cord stump	With diaper changes, rub alcohol on all sides of the umbilical stump and drip on some alcohol	Nearly always falls off by 3 weeks May be moist and green at the base Call doctor for erythema extending onto the abdominal skin or purulent discharge
Uncircumcised penis	Wash the penis with baths as you would other body parts	Do not forcibly retract the foreskin At age 1–2 years, gently retract or partially retract the foreskin weekly during the bath Never use soap beneath the foreskin Never leave the foreskin retracted after cleansing Contact your doctor if the foreskin does not retract by the age 18 years
Circumcised penis	Cleanse the area three times a day with water Petroleum jelly or Bacitracin may be applied after cleansing	The plasti-bell ring should fall off by 14 days Call the doctor if the glans becomes blue, black, red, or tender
Colic	Interventions to try: Carry the baby in an infant sling to increase contact Walk or rock with the baby Try an infant swing Ride in the car The sound of the vacuum cleaner or clothes dryer may be soothing In breastfeeding mothers, try eliminating milk, cabbage, or other potentially troublesome foods from mother's diet	The child usually cries for up to 3 hours at the same time each day Usually starts less than 2 weeks of age Usually stops by age 3 months

Metatarsus Adductus

Metatarsus adductus is a C-shaped curvature of the lateral border of the foot probably caused by the position of the foot *in utero* (Fig. 2.1). In 85% to 90% of cases the deformity resolves spontaneously by the age of 1 year, and little functional impairment is observed in those that do not, although treatment may be needed to facilitate fitting shoes. If the foot can be straightened when the heel is held firmly and the forefoot is abducted, a flexible deformity is present. If not, it is rigid. Treatment consists of stretching exercises, where the heel is stabilized and the forefoot is brought outward. This is repeated five times daily. Orthopedic referral for serial casting is indicated if the condition does not improve by 4 months; referral should be earlier if the deformity is rigid.

TABLE 2.5. Questions for day care providers

Ratio of children to staff (usually 6–8:1 for small children or 10–14:1 for older ones)
Are older and younger children separated (reduces risk of infection)?
Are policies written?
How are children disciplined?
Are staff members certified in first aid?
Are staff members trained in child development?
What are the hand-washing policies?
How and how often are toys cleaned?
Are outlet covers, smoke alarms, impact-absorbing playground surfaces used?
What happens if a child becomes ill?
What is a typical day like?

Adapted with permission from *American Family Physician* 1996. © 1996 American Academy of Family Physicians.

TABLE 2.6. Causes of failure to thrive

Psychosocial
Perinatal infection
Gastroesophageal reflux
Inborn errors of metabolism
Cystic fibrosis

Adapted with permission from Behrman RE, ed. *Nelson's textbook of pediatrics,* 15th ed. Philadelphia: WB Saunders, 1996:123.

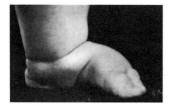

FIGURE 2.1. The diagnosis of metatarsus adductus is best made by observing the sole of the patient's foot. A C-shaped curve of the lateral border of the foot will be evident. (From Sponseller PD. Bone, joint, and muscle problems. In: McMillan JA, DeAngelis CD, Feigin RD, Warshaw JB, eds. *Oski's pediatrics: principles and practice.* Philadelphia: Lippincott Williams & Wilkins, 1999.)

DEVELOPMENTAL DYSPLASIA OF THE HIP

Developmental dysplasia of the hip occurs in approximately one per 1,000 newborns, with females and infants in breech presentation affected more often. Early diagnosis reduces the need for surgery and lessens the risk of persistent problems in the hip. The examination is performed with the child supine, the diaper off, and the hips and knees flexed to 90 degrees. On inspection, an unequal number of skin folds on one medial thigh compared with the other or an uneven level of the knees raise suspicion for a dislocated hip. In the Ortolani maneuver, the child is supine and the examiner's index and middle fingers are placed over the greater trochanter with the thumb along the medial thigh. The hip is then abducted and lifted anteriorly. If a "clunk" is felt as the hip reduces into the acetabulum, the test suggests a dislocated hip. In the Barlow maneuver, the examiner exerts posterior pressure on the knee while gently abducting the hip. The test suggests hip dislocation if a "clunk" is felt as the hip dislocates posteriorly out of the acetabulum (Fig. 2.2). Clicks (adventitial findings) in the hip may be a normal finding and may be difficult to distinguish from clunks. Ultrasound can be used to visualize the hips in the first few months of life before the hip is ossified. After 4 to 6 months, radiographs are useful. Dysplasia of the hip may present later in life, so even after a thorough initial evaluation, the examination should be repeated at office visits throughout the first year of life. If dysplasia is suspected, orthopedic referral is generally indicated for treatment, usually with a Pavlik harness or a Spika cast in the older child. Double or triple diapering is rarely indicated, as this may keep the hip in wide adduction, which increases the risk of avascular necrosis.

Management of other common medical problems is presented in Table 2.7.

REFERENCES

American Academy of Pediatrics, Section on Urology. Timing of elective surgery on the genitalia of male children with particular reference to the risks, benefits and psychological effects of surgery and anesthesia. *Pediatrics* 1996;97:590.

Committee on Ambulatory Quality Improvement. *Early detection of developmental dysplasia of the hip.* Elk Grove Village, Illinois: American Academy of Pediatrics, 2000.

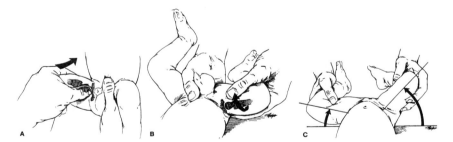

FIGURE 2.2. Barolow and Ortolani tests, performed with fingers on the lesser and greater trochanters, examining only one hip at a time. **A:** Barlow test: adduction and posterior pressure may produce a "clunk" of subluxation or dislocation. **B:** Ortolani test: abducting and "lifting" hip back into place. **C:** In children older than 3 to 6 months, Barlow and Ortolani tests often will be negative despite dislocation because of diminished laxity. The most important finding in this age group may be limitation of abduction. (From Sponseller PD. Bone, joint, and muscle problems. In: McMillan JA, DeAngelis CD, Feigin RD, Warshaw JB, eds. *Oski's pediatrics: principles and practice.* New York: Lippincott Williams & Wilkins, 1999.)

TABLE 2.7. Common medical problems in infants and young children

Problem	Intervention	Comments
Capillary hemangioma	Reassure parents	Lesions usually expand and then involute spontaneously
Decreased femoral pulses	Check blood pressure in all four extremities	Intervention only needed if lesion affects function (e.g., eyelid, urethra); 90% to 95% resolve by 9 years of age
Asymmetric red reflex	Refer to ophthalmologist	If blood pressure is less in legs than in arms, coarctation of the aorta must be ruled out
Corneal cloudiness	Refer to ophthalmologist	Could indicate cataract, retinal tumor
Subconjunctival hemorrhage	Reassure	Could indicate congenital glaucoma
Nasolacrimal duct obstruction	Massage upward over the lacrimal sac (inner lower corner of the eye) twice daily to remove secretions	Resolves spontaneously
		Usually present with excessive tearing or matter in the eye
		Children with a blocked duct are at increased risk of infection
		May need nasolacrimal duct probing by ophthalmologist if persists to age 6–12 months
		Topical antibiotics often required if drainage is purulent
Undescended testes	Reassure	Most testes descend spontaneously
		Urologic referral for orchidopexy recommended at age 1 year if testes not descended
Umbilical hernia	Reassure	Most resolve by age 1 year
		Strapping does not help
		Consider surgery if persists to age 3–4, symptomatic or enlarging after age 1 year
		Strangulation is very rare

Condition	Management	Notes
Inguinal hernia	Refer for operative repair	Does not resolve spontaneously Increased risk of incarceration in the first year of life
Hydrocele	Reassure	Nontender, can be transilluminated May increase in size with upright position Often resolves by 1 year of age If persists past 2 years of age urologic referral is indicated for management as for inguinal hernia Do not aspirate
Umbilical cord infection	Culture drainage Admit to hospital if child appears ill or infection appears severe Oral antibiotics, depending on culture results	Usually caused by group A strep or *Staphylococcus aureus* Can progress to serious infection
Pilonidal dimple	Reassure Encourage good hygiene	If deep or associated with a tuft of hair, consider ultrasound to rule out congenital spinal dermal sinus, which may extend to the intradural space

Ballock RT, Richards BS. Hip dysplasia: early diagnosis makes a difference. *Contemp Pediatr* 1997;14:108.

Bauchner H. Failure to thrive. In: Behrman RE, ed. *Nelson's textbook of pediatrics,* 15th ed. Philadelphia: WB Saunders, 1996:122.

Churgay C. Diagnosis and treatment of pediatric foot deformities. *Am Fam Physician* 1993;47:883.

Dietz FR. Intoeing: fact, fiction and opinion. *Am Fam Physician* 1994;50:1249.

Kapur P, Caty MG, Glick PL. Pediatric hernias and hydroceles. *Pediatr Clin North Am* 1998; 45:773.

O'Donnell KA, Glick PL, Caty MG. Pediatric umbilical problems. *Pediatr Clin North Am* 1998;45:791.

2-Month Visit

HISTORY

The 2-month visit occurs when infants are beginning to interact with their parents by smiling and cooing. Their care is still very demanding, but by this visit most parents have developed a routine. Ask about any illness or emergency visits. Also, particular attention should be paid to feedings, which consist exclusively of breast milk and/or formula at this age. Parents should be asked about concerns about diapers, diaper rash, stooling, and urinating. Children at this age sleep most of the time (greater than 16 hours daily is normal) but may awaken frequently at night. Parents should be asked about methods for putting the child to sleep and night-time awakenings. Finally, parents should be asked about new developmental abilities, any concerns about the child's development, and how the family is coping with the new addition, including signs of depression in the caregivers.

PHYSICAL EXAMINATION

The examination should begin by observing the infant during the history taking. How comfortable is the parent handling the child? The weight, length, and head circumference should be plotted on the growth chart. Observe the child for congenital malformations. The least invasive procedures (auscultation of heart) should be performed before the more invasive (otoscope). Particular areas of emphasis on the examination include the following:

Head—occipital flatness

Eye—red reflex, visual tracking

Heart—murmur

Abdomen—masses

Hips—dislocatability

Groin—femoral pulses

Perineum—diaper rash

Feet—metatarsus adductus

DEVELOPMENTAL MILESTONES

The two-month-old should be able to:

Hold his head temporarily erect

Briefly hold a rattle

Visually track and follow objects

Regard faces

Respond to sounds

Coo

Smile socially

If there is concern about development, a more complete evaluation, such as a Denver Developmental Screen should be performed, or referral should be made for a complete evaluation.

ANTICIPATORY GUIDANCE

Many parents of 2-month-olds become fatigued. Parents should arrange for time off, away from the child. Parents should be encouraged to rest when the child rests, especially if the child is awakening frequently. Many parents want to start solids at this age. They should be advised that the child cannot digest solids yet and should wait until age 4 months of age for solids. Expect on average one bowel movement daily if bottle feeding. Breastfed infants may stool from many times daily to once a week. If there are no signs of constipation and the child is growing well, all the preceding are considered normal. Many parents are concerned that their child is constipated. Constipation should be distinguished from normal straining, particularly as the child must move his bowels while on his back. If the stools are large and soft and there are no fissures, the caregiver should be reassured. In the formula-fed infant, changing brands of formula may help. Giving fruit juice such as prune juice or grape juice twice daily may help.

Sleep problems are common and can be very troublesome for new parents. Children should be put to sleep when drowsy yet awake so they can learn to fall asleep on their own. Parents should try to give the last feeding just before the parent goes to sleep. If the child awakens at night for a feeding, the feeding should be brief and boring. The child should not get in the habit of playing in the middle of the night. Breastfed infants often feed more during the night than bottle-fed infants. Many breastfeeding mothers keep the child with them and nurse on demand. This is particularly common if the mother is away during the day. If this is acceptable for the mother, it should not be discouraged. If the child sleeps more than 3 hours during the day, the caregiver should try to awaken the child.

Notice areas where the parents are excelling and praise them for this (Table 2.8).

TABLE 2.8. Anticipatory guidance at 2 months of age

Don't leave child where he can fall off; get ready for rolling over
Don't hold child and hot liquids; the child can spill them
Remember that playpens are an island of safety but don't use them too much
Remember that if it fits through a toilet paper roll, it's a choking hazard
Do not use walkers
Maintain a smoke-free environment
Avoid sun exposure
Expect four to six wet diapers daily
Talk to your child
Cuddle with your child
Always use the car seat
Do not give the child honey or corn syrup (botulism risk)

HEALTH MAINTENANCE

At this age a **hemoglobin or hematocrit** should be checked if the child was premature, had significant hemolysis, or experienced unusual blood loss. Many groups (The Joint Committee on Infant Hearing, The AAP, Bright Futures) recommend the goal of universal detection of infants with **hearing loss** as early as possible using brainstem or otoacoustic emissions. These screens can be performed from the newborn period through 3 months of age. The U.S. Preventive Services Task Force finds insufficient evidence to recommend for or against this routine screening. They do recommend screening in high-risk infants, including infants where there is caregiver concern, speech, language, or developmental delay, or a history in the family or child consistent with an increased risk of hearing loss.

Immunizations usually given at this age include IPV, DTaP, HiB, and hepatitis B. By federal law all providers are required to provide the Vaccine Information Sheets approved by the Centers for Disease Control (CDC) each time a vaccination is given. These are available from the CDC. The current immunization schedule is included in Appendix Table A.1. As this schedule is updated frequently, the provider should refer to the current American Academy of Family Physicians (AAFP) recommendations. To decrease the risk of fever and discomfort, many providers recommend that acetaminophen be given at the time of the immunization and 4 hours later. The acetaminophen dosing schedule is given in Appendix Table A.3.

MANAGEMENT OF COMMON MEDICAL PROBLEMS PRESENTING AT 2 MONTHS

With the increase in supine sleeping has come a decrease in sudden infant deaths, but concern over **misshapen heads** has increased. This problem is most common in infants who sleep on their backs, especially when they sleep in exactly the same position most of the time. Most often, the main risk is of a cosmetic deformity of the head. This defect becomes much less prominent as the child grows hair. Uncommon causes of a misshapen head include hydrocephalus, depressed skull fracture, intracranial tumor, and craniosynostosis (premature closure of a cranial suture) (Fig. 2.3). To lessen

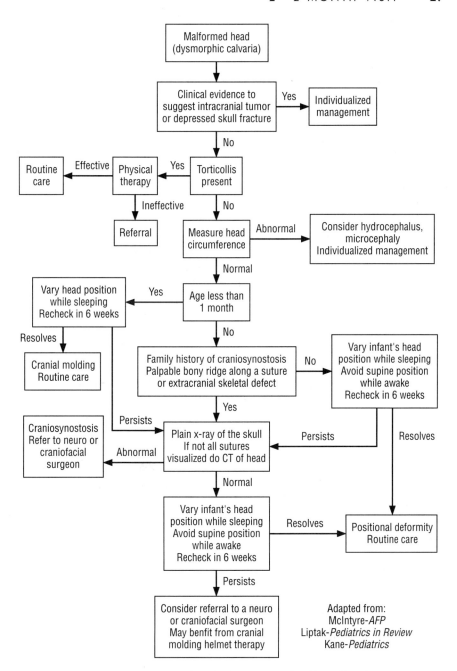

FIGURE 2.3. Algorithm for treatment of malformed head.

the risk of a misshapen skull, parents should vary the child's head position while the child is sleeping on his or her back and place the child both supine and prone while awake.

Diaper rash is common throughout infancy, although it is most common between 9 and 12 months of age. The frequency of diaper rash can be decreased by breastfeeding, frequent diaper changes, and the use of disposable diapers. Children with diarrhea are particularly prone to diaper rash. Caregivers should avoid excess scrubbing of the diaper area. After urination, no cleansing is usually needed, but after a bowel movement the area should be cleaned with a mild soap. Diaper wipes are convenient and usually well tolerated, but they may be irritating in the setting of dermatitis. Barrier creams, such as Balmex, A and D ointment, or Desitin, decrease contact between the skin and the urine and feces. Powders, especially corn starch, may reduce the friction and moisture. Corn starch does not increase the risk of candidiasis. Parents should keep powder away from the face to reduce the risk of aspiration. Table 2.9 lists the common causes of diaper dash and their treatment. Fluorinated and high-potency steroids, including those combined with anti-yeast preparations (Mycolog II, Lotrisone), should be avoided in the diaper area because of the risk of inflammation, striae, and adrenal suppression. If diaper rash is refractory to usual treatment, less common infections, including scabies, HIV, genital warts, such dermatoses as seborrheic dermatitis and psoriasis, or diabetes mellitus, should be considered.

REFERENCES

Arnsmeier SL, Paller AS. Getting to the bottom of diaper dermatitis. *Contemp Pediatr* 1997;14:115.

Kane AA, Mitchell LE, Craven KP, Marsh JL. Observations on a recent increase in plagiocephaly without synostosis. *Pediatrics* 1996;97:877.

Liptak GS, Serletti JM. Pediatric approach to craniosynostosis. *Pediatr Rev* 1998; 19:352.

McIntyre FL. Craniosynostosis. *Am Fam Physician* 1997;55:1173.

Singalavanij S, Frieden IJ. Diaper dermatitis. *Pediatr Rev* 1995;16:142.

U.S. Preventive Services Task Force. *Guide to clinical preventive services*, 2nd ed. Baltimore: Williams & Wilkins, 1996.

4-Month Visit

HISTORY

Healthy 4-month-olds are some of the most enjoyable patients seen in family practice. By this age the child can smile and is beginning to respond to parental interaction. Stranger anxiety is at a minimum. Parents are usually accustomed to the routine of caring for the child. Most new parents have multiple questions at this and all well-child visits. If none are asked, especially with first-time parents, the provider should probe deeper to verify parenting competence. Signs of parental stress, including concerns about child care, should be assessed. If solids have been offered to the child, the physician should ask how they are tolerated. Problems with bottle or breastfeeding, stooling, urination, sleeping, or night-time awakenings should be discussed. Parenting is a busy, full-time job, so coping skills of the parents as well as interaction with the extended family should be evaluated. Contraception should be reassessed.

TABLE 2.9. Common causes of diaper dermatitis

Irritant	Usual Age	Morphology	Distribution	Diagnosis	Treatment
Contact dermatitis	Peak 9–12 months; rare before 1 month	Erythema ± scaly, shallow ulcerations,	Convexities—buttock, thigh, abdomen, perineal area; spares, creases	Clinical	Hydrocortisone 1% four times daily. If rash presents for more than 3 days, add topical nystatin (Mycostatin), clotrimazole (Lotrimin), or ketoconazole (Nizoral) two times a day
Candidal diaper dermatitis	Any age	Beefy red, scaly plaques with satellites, papules, and pustules	Usually involves inguinal folds	Clinical KOH—pseudohyphae (may be negative if chronic)	Topical ketoconazole

Clotrimazole, nystatin two times daily. Add 1% hydrocortisone if significant inflammation is present |
| Bacterial infection | Any age | Crusts, vesicles, pustules, bullae | Anywhere—common in diaper area, periumbilical, suprapubic area | Clinical, gram stain, culture | Mupirocin (Bactroban) or Polysporin three times daily; cephalexin (Keflex) if extensive or bullous |
| Atopic dermatitis | Greater than 1 month | Erythema, papules, lichenification | Convex surfaces, worst area often adjacent to diaper | Clinical, often also present in other areas | Hydrocortisone 1% four times daily. Consider antistaphylococcal antibiotics when recalcitrant |

Adapted from Singalavanija S, Frieden IJ. Diaper dermatitis. Pediatr Rev 1995;16:142; and Arnsmeier SL, Paller AS. Getting to the bottom of diaper dermatitis. Contemp Pediatr 1997;14:115.

PHYSICAL

The physical examination begins with assessment of the parent/child interaction. At this age the child should smile readily. Abnormal facies may indicate that the child has a genetic syndrome and may require referral. Other areas of particular emphasis on the examination include the following:

Growth—weight, length, head circumference

Eyes—symmetric red reflex

Heart—murmur

Abdomen—masses

Hips—dislocatability

DEVELOPMENTAL MILESTONES

The 4-month-old should be able to:

Hold head erect

Raise body using arms

Roll over

Reach for objects, put hands together, grab a rattle

Visually track objects 180 degrees

Respond to sounds

Coo reciprocally, blow bubbles, raspberry

Smile readily in social situations, laugh or squeal, differentiate individuals

ANTICIPATORY GUIDANCE

Four-month-olds are more interactive than their younger counterparts. Nevertheless, their care can be fatiguing. Parents need to make time for themselves, even if they have competing demands with work and child care. Generally, solids can be started at this age. Infants who are ready for solids appear interested when other family members eat. They also do not thrust their tongues out when a spoon is placed in their mouth. If the child does thrust his tongue out, solids may be delayed for 1 to 2 weeks and tried again. Cereal should not be added to bottles unless there is a medical indication such as reflux. Parents need to realize that the solid food is mostly used for practice with eating solids. According to Mehta, children of this age still receive most of their nutrition from their breast milk or formula, and infants will displace energy needs from formula or breast milk as additional solids are consumed. In children with atopy or at high risk of atopy, solids may be delayed up to the age of 1 year, though if breastfed they will need iron supplementation at 4 to 6 months. Iron-fortified infant cereals are usually well tolerated and meet the iron needs of the breastfed infant. The order of introduction of other solids foods is arbitrary. Fruits, vegetables, and meats may be added in any order, but only one new food should be introduced every 3 days to facilitate identification of food intolerances. Combination products should be avoided until the individual components have been tolerated separately. Homemade pureed foods are nutritionally equivalent to commercially prepared ones. Excess sugar and salt should be avoided in either case. Honey may cause botulism in children younger than 1 year and so should be avoided. Juices may be introduced when the child can hold a cup and then limited to 8 ounces per day.

Other anticipatory guidance for this age includes the following:

Use a car seat whenever in the car.

Set the hot water heater at 120° to avoid scalding.

Avoid setting the baby on high places to decrease risk of falls.

Keep sharp objects out of the child's reach.

Do not drink hot liquids or smoke while holding the child to decrease burn risk.

Cover electrical outlets.

Remember that any object that can fit through a toilet paper roll poses a choking hazard.

Avoid baby walkers; use stationary spinners or jumpers instead.

Talk and read to the baby often.

COMMON MEDICAL PROBLEMS

Upper respiratory infections are common in young children (six per year on average, more in children attending day care). Mucopurulent nasal discharge is common in viral infections. Treatment is symptomatic, as antibiotics are not helpful. One method to clear the dry, stuffy nose is to instill 3 drops of warm water or saline into each nostril, wait 1 minute, then use a soft rubber suction bulb to clear the nostril. Parents should seek medical attention for wheezing, signs of dehydration, fever of more than 100°, or nasal congestion lasting more than 2 weeks. Studies have shown that decongestants (Pediacare) or combination decongestant and antihistamine products (Rondec, Triaminic) do not provide relief of nasal congestion, runny nose, or cough, although children given these products do tend to fall asleep sooner, probably because of the sedation of the antihistamine (Clemons). At times, prescribing these products may satisfy parents who had expected an antibiotic for their ill child.

Bronchiolitis is usually caused by the respiratory syncytial virus (RSV). Infection usually occurs in winter and is transmitted from direct contact or contact aerosolized droplets. The incubation period is 3 to 5 days. Breastfeeding is protective. The child usually begins with rhinorrhea and cough. The cough then becomes deeper, and in some children respiratory distress develops. A low-grade temperature, high-pitched wheezing with fine crackles, and hyperinflation of the chest are common. Children vary from having mild symptoms of upper respiratory infection to respiratory failure, with the latter being more common in young infants. The diagnosis may be confirmed through a nasal swab for the RSV antigen. Differentiation from acute asthma may be difficult, especially when a first episode of wheezing occurs in winter. For the mildly ill child, the management is supportive with hydration and antipyretics. Antibiotics are used only when there is concomitant bacterial infection such as otitis media. In general, steroids and inhaled bronchodilators are not effective for bronchiolitis, though they may be useful if there is coexisting bronchospasm. Severely ill children, with cyanosis or other signs of respiratory distress, require hospital admission. Recent trials have shown little to no benefit from the use of ribavirin, though it may be considered in very ill children, especially those with underlying illness (AAP, 1996). Children who have had bronchiolitis have an increased incidence of further wheezing, especially in the first 2 years after the illness. Prevention through good hand washing and decreased contact with infected persons is effective. Prophylactic, monthly, intramuscular injections of a monoclonal antibody against RSV, palivizumab (Synagis) has been shown to decrease the risk of severe RSV infection in certain children less than 24 months old with chronic lung disease (formerly named bronchopulmonary dysplasia) or prematurity.

HEALTH MAINTENANCE

Before giving this set of immunizations, discuss any adverse reactions from previous ones. Immunizations usually given at this age currently include IPV, DTaP, and Hib.

REFERENCES

American Academy of Pediatrics. Respiratory syncytial virus. In: Peter G, ed. *1997 Red Book: report of the Committee on Infectious Diseases*, 24th ed. Elk Grove Village, IL: American Academy of Pediatrics, 1997:443.

American Academy of Pediatrics, Committee on Infectious Diseases. Reassessment of indications for ribavirin therapy. *Pediatrics* 1996;97:137.

American Academy of Pediatrics, Committee on Infectious Diseases and Committee on the Fetus and Newborn. Prevention of respiratory syncytial virus infections: indications for the use of palivizumab and update on the use of RSV-IGIV. *Pediatrics* 1998;102:1211.

Clemons CJ, et al. Is an antihistamine-decongestant combination effective in temporarily relieving symptoms of the common cold in preschool children? *J Pediatr* 1997;130:501.

Hall CB, Hall WJ. Bronchiolitis. In: Hoekelman RA, ed. *Pediatric primary care,* 3rd ed. St Louis, MO: CV Mosby, 1997:1213.

Jeng M, Lemen RJ. Respiratory syncytial virus bronchiolitis. *Am Fam Physician* 1997;55:1139.

Mehta KC, et al. Trial on timing of introduction of solids and food type on infant growth. *Pediatrics* 1998;102:569.

Patient Education

Bronchiolitis in babies. Patient handout available online from AAFP at www.family-doctor.org.

6-Month Visit

HISTORY

Six-month-olds are increasingly interactive. They begin to show a preference for parents instead of strangers. Ask about feedings. Is the child tolerating solids? Are some foods not tolerated? Verify that the child is still on breast milk or formula, and reinforce that whole milk should be delayed until 1 year of age. Have the parents noticed crossing of the eyes? Can the child sit with support? Ask about problems with urination, moving bowels, or sleep. Discuss stresses in the family, and praise parenting strengths.

PHYSICAL EXAMINATION

The physical examination begins with assessment of the parent/child interaction. At this age the child should be able to sit and should have conjugate gaze. Have the

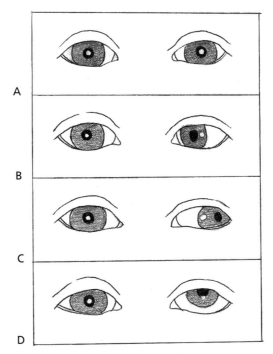

FIGURE 2.4. Findings during corneal light reflection. **A:** Normal alignment: the light reflections are centered on both corneas. **B:** Left esotropia: the light reflection is outwardly displaced on the left cornea. **C:** Left exotropia: The light reflection is inwardly displaced on the left cornea. **D:** Left hypertropia: The light reflection is downwardly displaced on the left cornea.

child follow a toy or other interesting object through all fields of vision. To do the corneal light reflex test (Hirschberg test) the examiner holds a light 3 feet from the child. The reflection of the light should fall in the same location within the pupil of each eye. The test should be repeated with the light in directions other than straight ahead. Figure 2.4 shows normal and abnormal results of the test. In pseudo-strabismus the eyes appear to deviate medially because of wide epicanthal folds (Fig. 2.5).

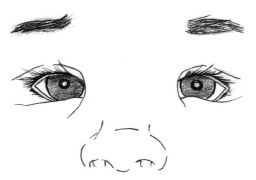

FIGURE 2.5. Pseudostrabismus resulting from a flat nasal bridge, wide epicanthal folds, and closely placed eyes. Note symmetric placement of the corneal light reflex (Hirschberg test).

If misalignment (strabismus) is suspected, the child should be referred to an ophthalmologist. Early treatment may prevent amblyopia (permanent visual impairment in the weak eye).

Other areas of particular emphasis on the examination include the following:

Growth—weight, length, head circumference

Eyes—conjugate gaze, symmetric red reflex

Heart—murmur

Abdomen—masses

Hips—dislocatability

DEVELOPMENTAL MILESTONES

The 6-month-old should be able to:

Hold his head high when prone, hold his head steady when pulled to sit, roll over, sit with support.

Obtain small objects with a raking movement.

Transfer objects.

Turn the head toward sounds and familiar voices.

Babble, laugh, and squeal.

Initiate social contact by smiling, cooing, laughing, and squealing.

Show pleasure and excitement with interactions with parents and others.

If there is concern about development, the child should undergo a more complete evaluation, such as a Denver Developmental Screen, or be referred for a more complete evaluation.

ANTICIPATORY GUIDANCE

Introduction of solids should be reviewed. A variety of foods, except junk foods, should be offered. Parental time off should be reemphasized. The child is becoming increasingly mobile, so the home must be child-proofed, including electrical outlets, sharp objects, and older children's toys.

Other anticipatory guidance may include the following:

Read to the child.

Limit TV.

Remember that plastic bags and household chemicals can be hazardous.

Set the hot water heater at less than 120°.

Provide safety around water, including the bathtub, toilet, and buckets.

Apply sunscreen (SPF 15 or greater with UVA and UVB protection) if sun exposure cannot be avoided.

Do not use a walker.

Remove guns from the home or keep them locked.

HEALTH MAINTENANCE

Currently recommended immunizations at 6 months of age are IPV, DTaP, HiB, hepatitis B.

COMMON MEDICAL PROBLEMS

Teething

Parents have multiple concerns about their children's teeth. Tooth eruption usually begins at 6 months of age. If teeth do not erupt before 1 year of age, the child may need evaluation by a dentist. If teeth are present in the first month of life, they need to be removed, because the normal tongue thrust during newborn swallowing will lead to tongue ulceration. Teething does not cause high fever, rash, or diarrhea, but many children do have mild irritability and mild temperature elevations. Massage of the gums or acetaminophen may help decrease discomfort. Chewing on a teething ring, Popsicle, teething biscuits, or frozen banana slices may help. Once teeth appear they may be cleaned with very small amounts of toothpaste on an infant toothbrush or, alternatively, with a damp cloth. To decrease the risk of caries, children should not go to bed with a bottle, and they should be weaned to a cup at 1 year of age. Breastfeeding mothers may be bitten by their teething child. Although many children never bite, pushing the child's face into the breast quickly teaches the child not to bite. Teething does not need to result in weaning, as most infants can be taught not to bite.

Fluoride

In areas with inadequate fluoride in the drinking water, fluoride supplementation should be considered. Fluoride supplementation recommendations are available from the AAP (Table 2.10). The fluoride concentration in the local water should be available from the Health Department. Care must be taken to avoid prescribing fluoride supplements to children with adequately fluoridated water. According to Clark, to decrease the risk of fluorosis, children should use only a pea-sized amount of toothpaste and not swallow it. With the increasing incidence of fluorosis and the increasing amount of fluoride found in children's foods and beverages, some authorities are recommending that fluoride supplements be limited to children at the highest risk of caries (Canadian Dental Association). Fluoride supplements are not needed for breast-fed infants in areas where the drinking water is fluoridated.

TABLE 2.10. Fluoride supplementation

Age	Water Fluoride Content (in ppm)		
	<0.3	0.3–0.6	>0.6
Birth–6 mo	0	0	0
6 mo–3 y	0.25	0	0
3–6 y	0.50	0.25	0
6–16 y	1.00	0.50	0

*Fluoride daily doses are given in milligrams.

Reprinted with permission from American Academy of Pediatrics, Committee on Nutrition: Fouoride Suplementation for Children: Interim policy recommendations. *Pediatrics* 1995;95:777.

Poisoning

As children become more mobile, the risk of poisonings increases. Medications should be kept out of reach and have child-proof caps. The number for the poison control center should be kept near the phone. Syrup of Ipecac should be kept in the home but not used except on the advice of the poison control center. The usual dose is 10 mL for children 6 months to 1 year, 15 mL for children more than 1 year of age but not yet adolescents, and 30 mL for adolescents. Ipecac should not be used in infants less than 6 months of age, patients with neurologic symptoms, and those with caustic or hydrocarbon ingestions. Parents should be asked what substance was ingested and told to bring the bottle for the poison to the emergency room with them. If the substance is nontoxic, parents may be reassured on the phone. Small, round objects pass spontaneously. Batteries are caustic and usually need to be removed.

Breath-Holding Spells

Breath-holding spells occur when the child is upset, such as after falling or being reprimanded. The child holds his breath in expiration, becomes bluish, and passes out. He then resumes normal breathing and is completely normal within 1 minute. These events may be difficult to distinguish from a seizure, and they often terrify parents. These spells do not lead to neurologic damage. Parents can be reassured and told to have the child lie flat during the spell. Parents should avoid overcomforting the child, as this positive reinforcement may lead to more frequent spells.

REFERENCES

American Academy of Pediatrics, Committee on Nutrition. Fluoride supplementation for children: interim policy recommendations. *Pediatrics* 1995;95:777.

Broderick P. Pediatric vision screening for the family physician. *Am Fam Physician* 1998;58:691.

Canadian Dental Association. Statement on fluoridation. Approved 9/98.

Clark MM, Album MM, Lloyd RW. Preventive dentistry and the family physician. *Am Fam Physician* 1996;53:619.

Nolan RJ. Poisoning. In: Hoekelman RA, ed. *Pediatric primary care.* St Louis, MO: CV Mosby, 1997:1738.

Patient Education

Strabismus. Handout from AAFP available online at www.familydoctor.org.

9-Month Visit

HISTORY

The 9-month-old is increasingly mobile. Parents may become fatigued with the effort required to keep the child constantly in sight. How does the child do with finger foods? Is the child still on breast milk or formula? Any concerns about stooling or urinating. When and how does the child go to sleep at night? Is she waking at night? Does she recognize her name, "no," "bye bye"? What do the parents do when the child misbehaves?

PHYSICAL EXAMINATION

At 9 months of age the child may be developing stranger anxiety. The examination may require more finesse, including examining the child on the parent's lap or pretending to examine the parent or a toy to decrease the child's discomfort. Check the teeth for discoloration or baby bottle caries. On neurologic examination the child should have a bilateral pincer grasp.

Other important aspects of the examination include the following:

Weight, length, head circumference

Strabismus, red reflex

Tooth eruption

Heart murmur

Abdominal masses

Hips

DEVELOPMENT

At 9 months of age the child should be able to:

Sit well, crawl, creep

Pick up small objects with thumb and index finger, feed self finger foods

Search for hidden objects, follow falling objects

Respond to name, wave bye-bye, babble in several syllables

Play peek-a-boo

Display the start of stranger anxiety

ANTICIPATORY GUIDANCE

At this age parents need to discipline their child. In general, it is often easier to remove objects that are not appropriate for the child than to try constantly to keep the child from them. When the child is seeking an inappropriate object, at this age he can often be easily distracted with another, appropriate object. Similarly, if the child is moving in an unwanted direction, the parent may be able to redirect her so she faces another way. The child may not remember the first objectives and so will be quite happy with the parent's selection. Spanking is quite controversial in the medical community but quite commonly used by parents. Children can be effectively disciplined without spanking, and in this way parents role-model nonviolent interaction. If spanking is used, the child may be spanked only with the hand, only on the buttocks, only so no marks are left, and only when the parent has good self-control.

Parents cannot talk too much to the child. One effective technique for the child to be exposed to speech is for the parent to tell the child everything the parent is doing. Spending the day with a small child is a learned skill. The caretaker should be praised whenever possible.

Children should remain in rear-facing car seats until they weigh 20 pounds and are 1 year old. Consistent use of cw seats prevents tantrums when the car is entered. Children of all ages are safest in the back seat and should never sit in a front seat with an enabled air bag. Figure 2.6 outlines the selection of car safety seats for children. Ide-

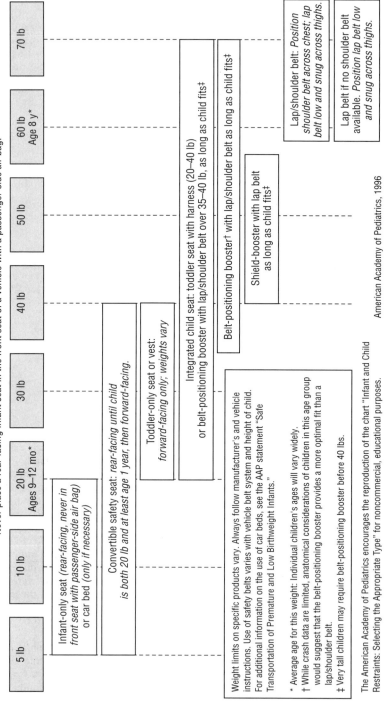

Infant and Child Restraints: Selecting the Appropriate Type

• The safest place for all children is the rear seat.
• Never place a rear-facing infant seat in the front seat of a vehicle with a passenger-side air bag.

| 5 lb | 10 lb | 20 lb
Ages 9–12 mo* | 30 lb | 40 lb | 50 lb | 60 lb
Age 8 y* | 70 lb |

Infant-only seat *(rear-facing, never in front seat with passenger-side air bag) or car bed (only if necessary)*

Convertible safety seat: *rear-facing until child is both 20 lb and at least age 1 year, then forward-facing.*

Toddler-only seat or vest: *forward-facing only; weights vary*

Integrated child seat: toddler seat with harness (20–40 lb) or belt-positioning booster with lap/shoulder belt over 35–40 lb, as long as child fits‡

Belt-positioning booster‡ with lap/shoulder belt as long as child fits‡

Shield-booster with lap belt as long as child fits‡

Lap/shoulder belt: *Position shoulder belt across chest; lap belt low and snug across thighs.*

Lap belt if no shoulder belt available. *Position lap belt low and snug across thighs.*

American Academy of Pediatrics, 1996

Weight limits on specific products vary. Always follow manufacturer's and vehicle instructions. Use of safety belts varies with vehicle belt system and height of child. For additional information on the use of car beds, see the AAP statement "Safe Transportation of Premature and Low Birthweight Infants."

* Average age for this weight: Individual children's ages will vary widely.
† While crash data are limited, anatomical considerations of children in this age group would suggest that the belt-positioning booster provides a more optimal fit than a lap/shoulder belt.
‡ Very tall children may require belt-positioning booster before 40 lbs.

The American Academy of Pediatrics encourages the reproduction of the chart "Infant and Child Restraints: Selecting the Appropriate Type" for noncommercial, educational purposes.

FIGURE 2.6. Selecting the appropriate type of car seat for infants and children. (Adapted with permission from *Infant and child restraints: selecting the appropriate type.* Elk Grove Village, Illinois: American Academy of Pediatrics, 1996.)

ally, the seat should be tried in the car before purchase, as different seats work best in different vehicles.

Other anticipatory guidance includes the following:

Praise parents

Offer a variety of foods

Minimize sibling rivalry

Eliminate choking hazards, such as hot dogs, peanuts, raw carrots, celery, popcorn

Child-proof the areas in which the child will be—remove sharp objects, watch out for older children's toys

Keep the water temperature below 120°

Provide safety around water

HEALTH MAINTENANCE

A hemoglobin should be checked in high-risk children, which includes children on whole milk, no-iron or low-iron formula, children living in poverty, African Americans, American Indians, Alaska Natives, immigrants from developing countries, and preterm or low-birth-weight infants. Because iron deficiency is overwhelmingly the most common cause of anemia in children, unless the history points to another cause, a therapeutic trial of iron supplementation may be instituted before additional workup. Table 2.11 lists common regimens for iron supplementation. Liquid iron supplements may stain teeth, so they should be given through a straw or with a dropper. Iron may cause constipation, dark stools, or abdominal cramping. The hemoglobin should be rechecked in 1 to 2 months. If no improvement is noted, additional workup is warranted.

TABLE 2.11. Iron supplements

Supplement	Dose	Concentration	Comments
Fer in Sol drops	6 mg/kg/day	15 mg/0.6 mL	
Fer in Sol syrup	6 mg/kg/day	18 mg/5 mL	
Feosol elixir	6 mg/kg/day	44 mg/5 mL	Give in three divided doses, 5% alcohol

REFERENCES

American Academy of Pediatrics. Committee on Injury and Poison Prevention. Selecting and using the most appropriate car safety seats for growing children: guidelines for counseling parents.

American Academy of Pediatrics, Committee on Psychosocial Aspects of Child and Family Health. Guidance for effective discipline. *Pediatrics* 1998;101:723.

Argan P, Winn D, Anderson C. Child occupant protection in motor vehicles. *Pediatr Rev* 1997;18:413.

U.S. Public Health Service. *Put prevention into practice: clinician's handbook of preventive services,* 2nd ed. International Medical Publishing, 1998.

Patient Education

Child behavior: what parents can do to change their child's behavior. Handout available from AAFP online at www.familydoctor.org.

1998 family shopping guide to car safety seats. AAP brochure. www.aap.org.

12-Month Visit

At the 12-month visit the child is often starting to walk, talk, and develop as an independent person. Discuss parental stress over the child's activity. Many parents notice decreased appetite after the first birthday. Formula may be replaced with whole milk at this age. For some this leads to constipation. Breastfeeding may be continued as long as mother and infant desire. Discuss concerns about stooling and urination. Is the child having temper tantrums? Discuss parents' plans for other children, and contraception, if applicable.

PHYSICAL EXAMINATION

At 12 months of age, playfulness by the examiner continues to facilitate the examination. Observe the parent/child interaction. How does the parent handle the child in the examination room? To minimize deterioration of undescended testes, orchiopexy is now recommended at 12 months of age.

Other important aspects of the physical examination include the following:

Weight, length, head circumference, weight for height

Strabismus, red reflex

Tooth eruption

Heart murmur

Testes

Leg alignment (see later)

Gait

DEVELOPMENT

At 12 months of age the child should

Sit without support, crawl, use pincer grasp, feed himself using a spoon or fingers.

Imitate adults, such as using a comb or telephone.

Display normal curiosity about genitals.

Play peek-a-boo and patty cake.

Imitate words.

Look at pictures in magazines.

ANTICIPATORY GUIDANCE

Praise parents.

Discuss sleep problems.

Take time out.

Child-proof appropriate areas—remove sharp objects, watch out for older kids' toys.

Provide bathroom safety.

Take time alone for parents.

Block stairs and doors.

Start toilet training at age 2.

Provide a bedtime routine.

Read to child.

Prevent the child from climbing dangerously.

Lock medications to prevent overdose.

Protect feet from injury and cold.

Change to whole cow's milk.

Provide pool safety.

HEALTH MAINTENANCE

Immunizations—HiB, measles–mumps–rubella (MMR), varicella

Tuberculin skin testing using the purified protein derivatives is recommended for high-risk children as defined in Table 2.12. Universal screening or screening with the tine test is no longer recommended. The test should be read by qualified health care personnel, not by the parents.

It should be repeated annually in HIV-infected children and every 2 to 3 years in other high-risk children. With the increasing prevalence of multidrug-resistant tuberculosis, children with a positive test for tuberculosis should generally be referred to specialists in the management of tuberculosis.

Blood lead screening is recommended if the child:

Lives in or regularly visits a house or day care facility built before 1950.

Lives in or regularly visits a house or day care facility built before 1978 that has been remodeled in the past 6 months.

Has a sibling or playmate with elevated lead levels.

TABLE 2.12.   Children at high risk for tuberculosis

Contacts of persons with confirmed or suspected tuberculosis
HIV-infected children
Contacts of persons in jail in the last 5 years
Children immigrating from endemic countries (Asia, Middle East, Africa, Latin America)
Children with travel to endemic countries or significant contact with persons indigenous to endemic countries
Children exposed to HIV-infected individuals, homeless persons, nursing home residents, institutionalized persons, migrant farm workers
Foster children with exposure to adults in the preceding groups

Used with permission from American Academy of Pediatrics. Tuberculosis. In: Peter G, ed. 1997 *Red book: report of the Committee on Infectious Diseases*, 24th ed. Elk Grove Village, IL: American Academy of Pediatrics, 1997:541.

TABLE 2.13. Techniques for accurate capillary lead sampling

Wear gloves
Wash the child's finger with soap and water
Cleanse area with alcohol
Wipe the first drop of blood off with sterile gauze and discard
Touch the drop of blood to the collection container
Do not allow the blood to flow under the nail
Once an adequate amount is collected, seal and agitate the specimen. If the lead level is elevated on a capillary sample, a venous level should be obtained. (Table 2.13 outlines the management of an elevated blood lead level.)

TABLE 2.14. Recommended follow-up services, according to diagnostic BLL

BLL (μg/dL)	Action
<10	No action required
10–14	Obtain a confirmatory venous BLL within 1 month; if still within this range,
	Provide education to decrease blood lead exposure
	Repeat BLL test within 3 months
15–19	Obtain a confirmatory venous BLL within 1 month; if still within this range,
	Take a careful environmental history
	Provide education to decrease blood lead exposure and to decrease lead absorption
	Repeat BLL test within 2 months
20–44	Obtain a confirmatory venous BLL within 1 week; if still within this range,
	Conduct a complete medical history (including an environmental evaluation and nutritional assessment) and physical examination
	Provide education to decrease blood lead exposure and to decrease lead absorption
	Either refer the patient to the local health department or provide case management that should include a detailed environmental investigation with lead hazard reduction and appropriate referrals for support services
	If BLL is >25 μg/dL, consider chelation (not currently recommended for BLLs <45 μg/dL), after consultation with clinicians experienced in lead toxicity treatment
45–69	Obtain a confirmatory venous BLL within 2 days; if still within this range,
	Conduct a complete medical history (including an environmental evaluation and nutritional assessment) and a physical examination
	Provide education to decrease blood lead exposure and to decrease lead absorption
	Either refer the patient to the local health department or provide case management that should include a detailed environmental investigation with lead hazard reduction and appropriate referrals for support services
	Begin chelation therapy in consultation with clinicians experienced in lead toxicity therapy
≥70	Hospitalize the patient and begin medical treatment immediately in consultation with clinicians experienced in lead toxicity therapy
	Obtain a confirmatory BLL immediately
	The rest of the management should be as noted for management of children with BLLs between 45 and 69 μg/dL

Used with permission from American Academy of Pediatrics. Committee on Environmental Health. Screening for Elevated Blood Lead Levels. *Pediatrics* 1998;101:1072–1078.

In communities where there is a high prevalence of elevated lead levels (>12%) universal screening is recommended. This prevalence should be available from the local health department. In general, capillary sampling is most convenient (Table 2.13).

If the lead level is elevated on a capillary sample, a venous level should be obtained. Table 2.14 outlines the management of an elevated blood lead level.

COMMON MEDICAL PROBLEMS

Intoeing

As children begin to walk, parents and grandparents frequently become concerned that the child is **intoeing,** or is "pigeon-toed." Some of this concern stems from the excessive medical treatment of these usually benign conditions in the past. If the child has pain, an abnormal neurologic examination, or a family history of rotational abnormalities that persisted into adulthood, early referral may be needed. **Internal tibial torsion** is usually first detected in the second year of life. As the child walks, the kneecaps point forward and the feet point inward (Fig. 2.7). In 95% of cases the condition resolves spontaneously and so parents may be reassured. Bracing had been used in the past but has not been shown to be effective. If the condition persists to 8 to 10 years of age, orthopedic referral should be considered. At this point, if the condition impairs function, tibial derotation osteotomy may be indicated.

Excessive femoral anteversion is the most common cause of intoeing; it too resolves spontaneously in 95% of children. It usually presents in early childhood, and these children walk with their patellae and feet pointing inward, with increased internal rotation of the hips (Fig. 2.8). Sitting in the "W" position with feet beside buttocks should be avoided, and exercises that emphasize external rotation such as ice skating and ballet should be encouraged. Splinting and shoe modification are ineffective. This condition rarely causes any functional limitation, though if it persists to age 8 to 10, orthopedic referral for possible derotation osteotomy should be considered.

Bow Legs and Knock Knees

Most children less than 3 years of age are bow legged, yet by age 5 they become knock-kneed, and adult alignment is achieved by 7 to 8 years of age. In most cases parents may be reassured that the child will outgrow the perceived problem. Figure 2.9 outlines the measurement of the deformity. Orthopedic referral is indicated if:

Stature is below the fifth percentile.

There is significant asymmetry.

Bow legs are worsening after the age of 2 years.

Knock knees are worsening after the age of 5 years.

There is a family history of pathologic conditions.

There are associated clinical abnormalities.

The intercondylar or intermalleolar distance is greater than 5 inches.

Flat Feet

Many infants and toddlers have flat feet. In most children the flat foot is flexible, meaning that they have an arch when non–weight-bearing and when standing tiptoe. This condition does not cause pain, and these children may be allowed to walk barefoot or in ordinary shoes or sneakers. Custom shoes or orthotics are not needed. Medial arch supports may help the adolescent who experiences foot fatigue after prolonged walking or athletics. Orthopedic referral is generally needed if the flat foot is not flexible.

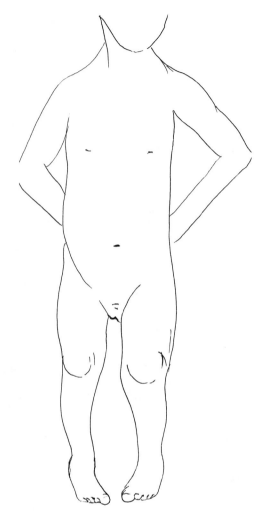

FIGURE 2.7. Intoeing caused by internal tibial torsion. The kneecaps point forward, while the feet point inward. The lateral border of the foot is straight.

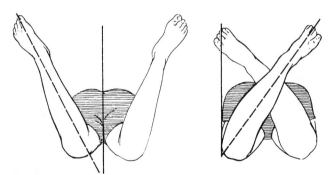

FIGURE 2.8. With the patient lying in a prone position and with the knees flexed 90°, the femurs are examined for their range of motion at the hips in extension. In excessive femoral anteversion, internal rotation is usually more than 70°.

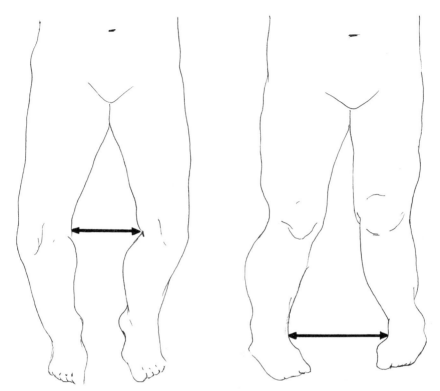

FIGURE 2.9. Knee bowing and knock-knees can be measured clinically. For bowing (left) the intercondylar distance (*arrow*) is measured with the ankles touching. In knock-knees (right) the intermalleolar distance (*arrow*) is measured with the knees together. A measurement of more than 5 to 6 inches suggests a severe condition requiring further evaluation.

REFERENCES

American Academy of Pediatrics. Committee on Environmental Health. Screening for elevated blood lead levels. *Pediatrics* 1998;101:1072.

American Academy of Pediatrics. Section on Urology. Timing of elective surgery on the genitalia of male children with particular reference to the risks, benefits and psychological effects of surgery and anesthesia. *Pediatrics* 1996;97:590.

American Academy of Pediatrics. Tuberculosis. In: Peter G, ed. *1997 Red Book: report of the Committee on Infectious Diseases*, 24th ed. Elk Grove Village, IL: American Academy of Pediatrics, 1997:541.

Bruce RW. Torsional and Angular Deformities. *Pediatr Clin North Am* 1996;43:867.

Churgay C. Diagnosis and treatment of pediatric foot deformities. *Am Fam Physician* 1993;47:883.

Dietz FR. Intoeing: fact, fiction and opinion. *Am Fam Physician* 1994;50:1249.

Mankin KR, Zimbler S. Gait and leg alignment: what's normal and what's not. *Contemp Pediatr* 1997;14:41.

Thompson GH, Scoles PV. The foot and toes. In: Behrman RE, ed. *Nelson's textbook of pediatrics*, 15th ed. Philadelphia: WB Saunders, 1996:1918.

Patient Education

Intoeing AAFP. Hanbdout available from AAFP online at www.familydoctor.org.

15-Month Visit

At age 15 months the toddler is quite mobile. What foods does the child eat? Has his appetite decreased? How much "junk" food is the child eating? Can the child drink from a cup? Are the parents weaning the bottle? Is the child aware of urinating or defecating? How is she sleeping? What new skills has the child learned? What do the parents do when the child misbehaves? How are temper tantrums handled?

PHYSICAL EXAMINATION

The physical examination may be increasingly difficult as the child becomes more independent. Particular areas of emphasis include the following:

Parent/child interaction

Weight, length, head circumference

Teeth

Heart murmur

Gait

Hernias

DEVELOPMENT

At 15 months of age the child should:

Feed self with fingers or spoon.

Scribble.

Pretend to use a toy phone.

Say single words.

Point.

Give and take toys.

Test parental limits.

ANTICIPATORY GUIDANCE

Although temper tantrums are a normal way for a young child to express anger and frustration, they can try the patience of even the best parent. During the tantrum children may cry, scream, bang their heads, hold their breath, slam doors, or throw things. If the child is in a safe environment, the tantrum should be ignored. If the child may break something or injure himself, he should be moved and then ignored. The parent cannot give in to the demands during the tantrum or the child will learn to use tantrums to manipulate caregivers. Even young children can be prepared for potentially difficult situations. For example, a parent might say, "If you behave in the store, we can play with your new truck when we get home." Potentially scary situations such as a doctor's visit can be explained ahead of time. Children are more prone to tantrums when they are tired, hungry, or ill, and so at these times stressful situations should be avoided when possible. If a child is having a tantrum due to fatigue or severe frustration, holding and comforting the child may calm him and end the tantrum. Children thrive on attention from adults, so if they receive abundant attention for good behavior, they are less likely to use bad behavior to gain attention. Also, children model their behavior on that of adults, so adults should try to control their own anger and avoid their own "tantrums."

Other anticipatory guidance includes the following:

Praise for parents

Child proofing (removal of sharp objects, watching out for older children's toys)

Bike helmets

Lowering of the crib mattress

Time alone for parents

Blocking of the stairs and doors

Toilet training at age 2

Consistent bedtime routine

Reading to child

Avoidance of dangerous climbing

Locking up of medications

Removal of plastic bags (suffocation hazard)

HEALTH MAINTENANCE

DTaP

COMMON MEDICAL PROBLEMS

The child with **croup** presents with a characteristic barking or seal-like cough, often preceded by nasal congestion. Narrowing in the subglottic region results in inspiratory stridor, which is associated at times with use of accessory muscles for respiration. On auscultation the child has a prolonged inspiratory phase that may be accompanied by wheezes or rhonchi. Aspiration of a foreign body may also present with cough and stridor, so this may need to be ruled out, depending on the history and clinical course. As the origin of croup is nearly always viral, antibiotics are not beneficial. Exposure to cool mist from a nebulizer or vaporizer, or cool night air may decrease the spasm and lead to rapid clinical improvement. In moderately severe croup, steroids have been shown to result in more rapid clinical improvement than placebo (Johnson, Klaussen). The usual dose is dexamethasone 0.6 mg/kg given once either orally or intramuscularly. Nebulized racemic epinephrine 0.05 mL/kg may be beneficial. (If racemic epinephrine is unavailable, epinephrine 1:1,000, 0.5 mL/kg may be substituted.) In the past, all children given racemic epinephrine were admitted to the hospital, but current recommendations are to observe the child for 1 to 3 hours and discharge home with close follow-up if the child does not have stridor or retractions (Knapp). Table 2.15 lists indications for admission.

T ABLE 2.15. Indications for hospital admission of patients with croup

Toxic appearance
Diagnosis of respiratory distress is uncertain
Restlessness
Changed sensorium
Oxygen requirement

REFERENCES

Johnson DW, et al. A comparison of nebulized budesonide, intramuscular dexamethasone, and placebo for moderately severe croup. *N Engl J Med* 1998;339:498.

Klaussen TP, et al. Nebulized budesonide and oral dexamethasone for the treatment of croup: a randomized controlled trial. *JAMA* 1998;279:1629.

Knapp JF. What's new in pediatric emergency medicine. *Pediatr Rev* 1997;18:424.

18-Month Visit

HISTORY

The 18-month-old continues to develop independence. The child should be able to express desires using words. Discuss the child's appetite. Any interest in the potty? What new things can the child do? Any behavioral problems? What do the caregivers enjoy most about the child? How are the caregivers coping with the child? How is the family getting along together?

PHYSICAL EXAMINATION

On physical examination pay particular attention to:

Parent/child interaction

Weight, length, head circumference

Teeth

Gait

Inguinal hernia

DEVELOPMENT

The 18-month-old

Walks up stairs with one hand held.

Stacks blocks.

Plays at pretend games.

Understands commands.

Likes to play with other children.

ANTICIPATORY GUIDANCE

By the time a child is 18 months old, many parents begin to be interested in **potty training,** although the child may not be. Most children are ready for toilet training at age 2, although this age varies widely. The first step is to place a potty in a room where the child plays. At first the parents should not mention or encourage any use of the potty. This allows the child to become accustomed to seeing it. Then the child may be encouraged to sit on the potty with clothes on. This time is ideal for reading or singing to the child. As the potty experience needs to be positive, the child cannot be forced. Meanwhile the child should observe adults or siblings using the bathroom and should learn the words for urinating and stooling. Once the child is accustomed to the potty, the parent may encourage her to sit on the potty with pants off, especially when the parents notice signs of needing to defecate or urinate. If the child does urinate or defecate in the potty, the parent should give generous positive reinforcement. If the process is not effective or becomes frustrating, the parent should stop all efforts and retry in a few weeks. Negative reinforcement is not effective and frequently leads to constipation rather than toilet training. Special rewards given only for use of the potty can be very effective. Parents should expect accidents and try to keep positive. Toilet training should not be attempted at times of increased family stress, when the child is ill, or if the child is unwilling.

Thumb sucking at this age is a normal self-comforting response. If the thumb-sucking occurs when the child is bored, he may be distracted. Overall, children rarely continue to suck the thumb past 4 years of age, unless the parents become overly concerned and cause a power struggle.

Other anticipatory guidance includes the following:

Praise for parents

Offering of healthy snacks

Weaning from the bottle

Watchfulness for excess sugar, salt, and fat

Children rarely share at this age

Time alone for parents

Blocking of stairs and doors

Bedtime routine

HEALTH MAINTENANCE

Verify that all the childhood immunizations are up-to-date. If a child is behind on the immunization schedule, the schedule for children not immunized in the first year of life should be consulted, because in some cases not all the vaccinations in the usual series are needed (Table 2.16).

T ABLE 2.16. Recommended immunization schedules for children not immunized in the first year of life*

Recommended Time/Age	Immunization(s)†‡§	Comments
Younger Than 7 Years		
First visit	DTaP, Hib, HBV, MMR, IPV	If indicated, tuberculin testing may be done at same visit
		If child is 5 years of age or older, Hib is not indicated in most circumstances
Interval after first visit		
1 month (4 weeks)	DTaP, HBV, Var#	The second dose of IPV may be given if accelerated poliomyelitis vaccination is necessary, such as for travelers to areas where polio is endemic
		Second dose of Hib is indicated only if the first dose was received when younger than 15 months
2 months	DTaP, Hib, IVP	IPV and HBV are not given if the third doses were given earlier
≥8 months	DTaP, HBV, IPV	DTaP is not necessary if the fourth dose was given after the fourth birthday;
Age 4–6 years (at or before school entry)	DTaP, IPV, MMR**	IPV is not necessary if the third dose was given after the fourth birthday.
Age 11–12 years	Td	
7–12 Years		
First visit	HBV, MMR, Td, IPV	
Interval after first visit		
2 months (8 weeks)	HBV, MMR,** Var,# Td, IVP	IPV also may be given 1 month after the first visit if accelerated poliomyelitis vaccination is necessary.

| 8–14 months | HBV,[††] Td, IPV | IPV is not given if the third dose was given earlier |
| Age 11–12 years | Td | |

Vaccine abbreviations: HBV indicates hepatitis B virus vaccine; Var, varicella vaccine; DTP, diphtheria and tetanus toxoids and pertussis vaccine; DTaP, diphtheria and tetanus toxoids and acellular pertussis vaccine; Hib, *Haemophilus influenzae* type b conjugate vaccine; IPV, inactivated poliovirus vaccine; MMR, live measles-mumps-rubella vaccine; Td, adult tetanus toxoid (full dose) and diphtheria toxoid (reduced dose), for children ≥7 years and adults.

*Table is not completely consistent with all package inserts. For products used, also consult manufacturer's package insert for instructions on storage, handling, dosage, and administration. Biologics prepared by different manufacturers may vary, and package inserts of the same manufacturer may change from time to time. Therefore, the physician should be aware of the contents of the current package insert.

†If all needed vaccines cannot be administered simultaneously, priority should be given to protecting the child against those diseases that pose the greatest immediate risk. In the United States, these diseases for children younger than 2 years usually are measles and *Haemophilus influenzae* type b infection; for children older than 7 years, they are measles, mumps, and rubella. Before 13 years of age, immunity against hepatitis B and varicella should be ensured.

‡DTaP, HBV, Hib, MMR, and Var can be given simultaneously at separate sites if failure of the patient to return for future immunizations is a concern.

#Varicella vaccine can be administered to susceptible children any time after 12 months of age. Unvaccinated children who lack a reliable history of chicken pox should be vaccinated before their 13th birthday.

**Minimal interval between doses of MMR is 1 month (4 weeks).

††HBV may be given earlier in a 0-, 2-, and 4-month schedule.

Used with permission from Peter G, ed. *1997 Red book: report of the Committee on Infectious Diseases,* 24th ed. Elk Grove Vilage, Illinois: American Academy of Pediatrics, 1997:1.

REFERENCES

American Academy of Pediatrics. Active and passive immunization. In: Peter G, ed. *1997 Red Book: report of the Committee on Infectious Diseases*, 24th ed. Elk Grove Village, IL: American Academy of Pediatrics; 1997:1.

Schmidt BD. *Your child's health.* New York: Bantam, 1991.

2-Year Visit

HISTORY

At the age of 2 years children are very mobile. They test limits imposed by caregivers and express themselves with words. They frequently run to the parent's lap when the physician enters the room and resist new caregivers. Discuss the child's diet. Children of this age may decide to eat a certain food repeatedly for a few days and then change to another food. Over time they tend to eat a balanced diet if one is offered. Parents may also note a decrease in appetite. As long as the child is growing well and is eating healthy foods, the parent can be reassured. Does the child use a cup? Does he sit at the table? Is the child using the potty? Are there any problems with elimination? How is the child sleeping? Does he awaken at night? What new activities can he do? How are the parents coping with the child?

PHYSICAL EXAMINATION

Discuss any physical concerns the parent may have. On the examination pay particular attention to:

Parent/child interaction

Weight, length, head circumference

Teeth

Leg alignment

Hernias

DEVELOPMENT

The 2-year-old child should

Walk up and down stairs.

Open a door.

Engage in early pretend play.

Have a vocabulary of greater than 50 words.

Follow two-step commands.

Brush teeth with help.

Feed herself.

ANTICIPATORY GUIDANCE

Discipline becomes increasingly important for the parents of toddlers. Good discipline begins with the parent giving reinforcement for good behavior. It may be quite difficult for the busy parent to stop and praise the child who is playing quietly, but this is essential. Parents need to make time to interact with their children, or the children will demand attention at the most inconvenient times. Parents also need to have developmentally appropriate expectations. A 2-year-old will not sit quietly for 2 hours. Parents need to anticipate the child's needs and bring toys if prolonged waiting is expected. Children should be offered acceptable choices when possible. For example, the parent might say, "Would you like to clean up your toys or put on your pajamas first?"

Another technique that works well at this age is removing the offending object. For example, if the child is hitting with a toy or two children are fighting over a toy, it should be taken away. Children quickly learn that they will lose desired objects if they do not follow the rules.

Time out is a very effective method of disciplining children. If the child misbehaves, he is sat down for 1 minute for each year of age. For young children, strapping them into a car seat or high chair works well. Some very resourceful children will need to be held in place as they become accustomed to time out. If the child screams, the timer is not started until the child is quiet. During time out the parent should ignore the child, while verifying that the child is still in time out. When the time is completed the parent allows the child up and should try not to remain angry with the child. Parents cannot threaten time out and not implement it, or the child will constantly test the parent. If the parent is consistent in implementation, simply telling the child that he will receive time out if he does not comply will often stop undesired behavior. Parents need to choose their battles and only punish for definite misbehavior; some small infractions can be overlooked. Many parents claim that their child will not do time out. In this case carefully review their technique. In most instances the parents have not been persistent in implementing the technique. Barton Schmidt's parenting textbook gives many details on time out and other discipline techniques.

Sleep problems are common in toddlers and children. In general, prevention is easier than treatment. Children should have a consistent bedtime and routine. The usual routine lasts 30 minutes and consists of a bath, tooth brushing, toileting, and a soothing bedtime story. Children should fall asleep in their beds so that if they reawaken during the night, they recognize their surroundings. If the child awakens at night, he can be briefly calmed and returned to bed. Parents should clearly state the expectation that the child stay in his own bed until daytime and praise him when he does. At this age the child can usually climb out of the crib; therefore the child should now sleep in a bed. Children of this age cannot be safely allowed to roam the house when the adults are asleep, and so the child may need to be gated in the room or furniture placed so he will make noise if he tries to leave his room. **Nightmares** are frightening dreams that awaken the child. The parent should comfort the child and reassure him of his safety. A night light may help. During the day the parent should discuss the dream and again reassure the child. Exposure to frightening situations, including videos and television shows, should be eliminated. Parents should verify that the nightmares are not signs of unusual stress in the child's life. **Night terrors** occur during deep sleep. The child is agitated and often screams. Since the child is still asleep, he cannot be comforted, and the child may even be afraid of the parent. The parent should keep the child from harm and try to calm him into usual sleep. In the morning the child does not recall the episodes. Avoiding overtiredness may help.

Other anticipatory guidance includes the following:

Praise for parents

Infant/toddler car seats, which are safer than booster seats

Healthy food choices

Children rarely share at this age

Climbing can be dangerous

Time alone for parents

Door Safety

Reading to child

Locking up of medications

Limitation of TV time

HEALTH MAINTENANCE

Verify that immunizations are up-to-date.

COMMON MEDICAL PROBLEMS

In the United State **obesity** is epidemic. Parents should take steps to avoid increasing their child's weight, usually beginning at age 2. Table 2.17 lists tips for parents.

REFERENCES

Moran R. Evaluation and treatment of childhood obesity. *Am Fam Physician* 1999;59(4):861.

Schmitt BD. *Your child's health.* New York: Bantam Books, 1991.

Patient Education

Child behavior: what parents can do to change their child's behavior. Handout available from AAFP online at www.familydoctor.org.

T ABLE 2.17. Tips for preventing obesity

Respect the child's appetite; do not require children to clean their plates
Keep high-sugar and high-fat foods out of the home
Keep ample fiber in the diet
Make healthy snacks such as fruit, vegetables, or raisins available
Change to skim or 1% milk at age 2 years
Do not use food for comfort or as a reward
Limit TV and video viewing
Encourage active play
Establish active activities for the whole family—for example, walking, hiking, swimming
Set a good example by exercising and eating a healthy diet yourself

Adapted with ermission from Moran R. Evaluation and treatment of childhood obesity. *Am Fam Physician* 1999;59(4):861.

Preschool Visit

HISTORY

Every child should have an office evaluation at the age of 3 or 4 years. Obviously, in children with ongoing medical or social issues, more frequent visits are needed. At this visit the child can often participate in the history, and this participation should be encouraged. Ask about illnesses, accidents, or other health concerns. How is the child's appetite? What foods does he eat? Is he using a spoon and fork? What new skills has he acquired? Is he sleeping through the night, in his own bed? How is the potty training going? Are there behavioral concerns?

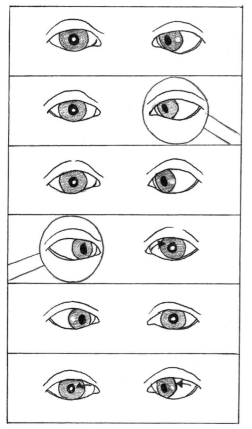

In a child with esotropia, one eye is deviated inward. Note that the corneal light on that eye is not centrally placed.

When the esotropic eye is covered, there is no movement of either eye. The uncovered eye maintains fixation.

The cover is removed. There is no movement of either eye.

When the other eye is covered, the previously esotropic eye takes up fixation and the covered eye turns inward (becomes esotropic) under the cover.

If the cover is removed and no eye movement occurs, an absence of a strong preference is suggested. Both eyes have approximately equal vision. The diagnosis is alternating strabismus, associated with a lower risk of amblyopia.

If the cover is removed and both eyes move back to their original positions (the originally esotropic eye is again esotropic), there is a fixation preference by one eye. This indicates a monocular strabismus. The esotropic eye is at righ risk for amblyopia. The same maneuvers can be used to determine the presence of exotropia (outward deviation), hyper- and hypotropia (upward and downward deviation), and cyclotropia (rotary displacement).

FIGURE 2.10. Monocular and intermittent strabismus as demonstrated by cover/uncover testing. (Adapted from Broderick P. Pediatric Vision Screening for the Family Physician. *American Family Physician* 1998;58:691–702.)

PHYSICAL EXAMINATION

At 3 years of age the routine physical examination should include measurement of blood pressure, which should be recorded with a cuff that covers two thirds of the distance between the shoulder and antecubital fossa. In general, a cuff that is too large is better than one that is too small, since measurement with one that is too small can lead to overestimation of the systolic blood pressure. (Table 5 in the Appendix gives the classification of hypertension in children.) At this age the AAFP recommends that the child be screened for amblyopia and strabismus. To do the cover/uncover test the child focuses on an interesting object 10 feet away. The physician then covers one eye with a cupped hand or an occluder. Figure 2.10 shows the interpretation of the examination. Visual acuity may be tested using a picture chart or the "Tumbling E" method.

Other aspects of the physical examination include the following:

Height and weight

Subjective hearing evaluation

Gait, leg alignment, hip rotation

Signs of abuse

DEVELOPMENT

During the preschool visits assessment of development is crucial. These visits occur infrequently, and yet early detection of developmental abnormalities is associated with improved outcome. In most areas referral sources for more complete developmental assessment are available if the physician suspects developmental issues.

At 3 years of age the child:

Exhibits bowel and usually bladder control.

Asks questions (why?).

Rides a tricycle.

Copies a circle.

Has 75% intelligible speech.

Engages in parallel play with other children.

At age 4 years the child:

Recognizes colors.

Copies a cross and square.

Speaks in phrases.

Hops on one foot.

Engages in role playing.

ANTICIPATORY GUIDANCE

Each year 150,000 children are injured on **playgrounds** in the United States. To minimize these injuries caregivers can

Remove drawstrings from hoods.

Verify that elevated surfaces have chest high guard rails.

Remove hazards such as rocks and broken glass.

Verify a 6-foot zone covered with a soft mulch or sand surrounding play equipment.

Allow children to play on age-appropriate equipment in the way it was intended.

Supervise young children.

Notify authorities of damaged equipment.

Sleepwalking is a condition in which the child walks or performs semipurposeful acts while asleep. The child usually appears dazed and does not answer questions. Parents should be reassured that these spells are not harmful to the child. The child should be led back to bed, protected from harm, and not awakened.

Thumb sucking is a common method for young children to comfort themselves. By the preschool years most children stop. Some continue. Once the permanent teeth come in, usually age 5 or 6, thumb sucking may be a risk factor for an overbite. To stop thumb sucking, convince the child he wants to stop. For example, mention that older children do not suck their thumbs, or show the child the callus on the thumb. Then give positive reinforcement for not thumb sucking at times he usually would. If the child wants help, an over-the-counter bitter medication can be applied to the thumb as a reminder, or a bandage or glove can be applied to the thumb at night. Negative reinforcement such as punishment or scolding is unlikely to be effective.

Nail biting is also common and is seen in nearly one fourth of normal young children, especially in times of stress. Possible complications include damage to the nail, infection, or dental problems. Methods of stopping nail biting are similar to those for stopping thumb sucking. First convince the child he wants to quit. Then give positive reinforcement for allowing the nails to grow. If the child desires, a bitter medication can be applied to the nails as a reminder.

Other anticipatory guidance includes the following:

Bedtime ritual

Talking to your child

Family meals

Limiting TV

Bike helmets

Gun safety

HEALTH MAINTENANCE

A first dental visit is generally recommended at 3 years of age.

COMMON MEDICAL PROBLEMS

Family physicians treat many children who are at risk because of poor family support, lack of educational opportunities, poverty, or other problems. For many of these children participation in an early intervention program can improve school success. Family physicians can make families aware of programs such as Head Start and encourage the child and family's participation.

REFERENCES

Broderick P. Pediatric vision screening for the family physician. *Am Fam Physician* 1998;58:691.

Foster LG. Nervous habits and stereotyped behaviors in preschool children. J Am Acad Child Adolesc Psychiatry 1998;37:711.

Haber JS. Early diagnosis and referral of children with developmental disabilities. *Am Fam Physician* 1991;43:132.

Leung AK, Robson WL. Nailbiting. *Clin Pediatr* 1990;29:690.

Kindergarten Visit

HISTORY

The kindergarten visit occurs at a time of excitement in the family. Entering school is a milestone in the child and parent's life. Begin the interview by talking with the child. Ask about friends and activities. Once the child is comfortable talking, ask about any illness or other concerns. Ask parents about their concerns regarding school entry. Who will be providing child care after school? Does the parent have any concerns? What is the child eating? Any toileting problems? Any sleep problems? What new skills has the child learned? How is the child disciplined? Does the child wear a bike helmet and seat belt?

PHYSICAL EXAMINATION

At this age the child has increased modesty.
    On examination pay particular attention to the following:

Height/weight/blood pressure

Strabismus

Visual acuity—Snellen chart

Subjective hearing evaluation

Gait, leg alignment, hip rotation

Signs of abuse

DEVELOPMENT

Once the child enters school, the school usually monitors the child's development. The parent may be asked about the child's school progress and if the child is receiving or needs special services. The parent should discuss any developmental concerns.
    The 5-year-old should be able to

Hop and climb on the examination table.

Copy squares, triangles.

Count to 10.

Name four colors.

Follow simple directions.

ANTICIPATORY GUIDANCE

Many parents are concerned about their child's readiness for school. A recent study has found that children who are older than their classmates have greater behavioral problems than their peers, even children without a history of being held back in school (Byrd). Families should be made aware of these findings if they are considering delaying school entry.

At the age of 4 or 5 years many states no longer require car seats for children. Many parents misinterpret this to mean that the child is safe in an adult seat belt. Many shoulder belts cross the child's neck and are unsafe. Children are safest in the back seat, in a belt positioning booster seat or an integrated child safety seat.

If a permanent is tooth knocked out and is intact, it should be rinsed and replaced in the socket. If replacement is impossible, the tooth can be transported in cool water or milk. In either case the dentist should be consulted immediately. Primary teeth should not be reinserted. Once the permanent molars are in, the parents should consult the dentist about the need for dental sealants.

Other anticipatory guidance includes the following:

Bedtime ritual

Talking to your child

Family meals

Limitation of TV

Positive reinforcement

Teaching children about 911

Chores that teach responsibility

Car safety

Limitation of junk food

HEALTH MAINTENANCE

Usual immunizations at this age include DTaP, IPV, MMR.

Tuberculin skin testing is indicated in

Children whose parents (with unknown tuberculin skin test status) immigrated from regions of the world with high prevalence of tuberculosis

Children who reside in areas with a high prevalence of tuberculosis (public health officials can identify high-risk neighborhoods or blocks)

COMMON MEDICAL PROBLEMS

Head lice are common in the school-aged child. Parents are universally embarrassed, but lice are not a reflection of poor hygiene. Some children present with pruritus, but many are asymptomatic. Transmission is usually by hair-to-hair contact, with transmission via fomites such as hats or combs being controversial. Lice do not have wings and cannot jump from person to person. Diagnosis is made by detecting live lice or eggs and is facilitated by adequate lighting, a magnifying glass, and a nit comb. Eggs are usually found close to the scalp and are distinguished from other scalp debris by their firm attachment to the hair shaft.

T ABLE 2.18.   Medications for the treatment of head lice

Medication	Application Instructions	Comments
Permethrin 1% (Nix)	Use as a cream rinse after washing the hair Rinse after 10 minutes	Allergic contact dermatitis can occur
Permethrin 5% cream (Elimite)	Leave on overnight under a shower cap	Only anecdotal reports of efficacy May not be more effective than the 1% formulation
Pyrethrin (Rid)	Apply to dry hair for 10 minutes, then rinse and shampoo or condition	2 ounces per application for up to medium-length hair

Follow package inserts for detailed instructions.
All treatments must be repeated in 7–12 days to eradicate newly hatched nymphs.
Products are best rinsed in the sink instead of the shower to limit exposure.
Following treatment, a nit comb should be used to remove eggs.

Adapted from Burgess IF. Lice: resistance and treatment. *Contemp Pediatr* 1998;15:181; and Chesney PJ. Drugs for head lice. *Med Lett* 1997;39:992.

Treatment, which may be frustrating, begins with application of a pediculicide, usually 1% permethrin (Nix) or pyrethrin (Rid) (Table 2.18). Because of concerns about neurotoxicity, especially with misuse, lindane should usually be avoided. After the treatment, lice and eggs are mechanically removed with a metal nit comb. The caregiver should begin at the scalp and work outward, washing the comb frequently, often with an old toothbrush. When possible, the comb should be moved along the hair toward the scalp, as this tends to loosen the egg from the hair shaft. This process is time-consuming, especially with long hair. Application of a 1:1 mixture of water and vinegar may loosen the egg's glue. The pediculicide should be repeated in 7 to 12 days to eradicate any newly hatched nymphs that may have survived in the egg during the first treatment. All close contacts of the infected child should be inspected closely for infection, but only those with evidence of infection should be treated, as prophylaxis is ineffective. Because the louse is specific for a human host, it cannot be carried on pets. Resistance to pediculicides is becoming more common, especially in children who have been previously treated. In resistant cases, treatment with 5% permethrin (Elimite) or trimethoprim sulfamethoxazole (Bactrim, Septra) (8 mg/kg/day of trimethoprim divided into two doses for 10 days) has been anecdotally effective. Ivermectin (Stromectol), 200 μg/kg orally and repeated once in 10 days, may be another option. A dense application of olive oil or mayonnaise beneath a shower cap overnight may suffocate the lice. Application of flammable substances such as kerosene is dangerous and should be avoided.

Environmental cleansing may not be needed because away from the human host, lice quickly become malnourished. Nevertheless, most authorities recommend cleaning towels and bedding by placing them in the dryer on high heat for 20 minutes and then laundering in regular detergent. Other objects may be placed in plastic bags for 2 weeks. As the lice must eat from the host every 4 to 6 hours, they die under these conditions. In freezing weather the bags may be placed outside overnight. Furniture and carpets should be vacuumed to remove loose hairs. Chemical extermination is not helpful.

Return to school is controversial. Some argue that the child should be nit-free before returning. Others argue that as lice are unpleasant but not medically harmful, the risk to other children is minimal once a child has been treated. Also distinguishing nits from other scalp debris can be quite difficult. Often these decisions are left to the school policy makers.

REFERENCES

Byrd RS, Weitzman M, Auninger P. Increased behavior problems associated with delayed school entry. *Pediatrics* 1997;100:654.

Chesney PJ, Burgess IF. Lice: Resistance and treatment. *Contemp Pediatr* 1998;15:181.

Drugs for head lice. *Med Lett* 1997;39:992.

Pollack RJ, et al. Differential permethrin susceptibility of head lice sampled in the United States and Borneo. *Arch Pediatr Adolesc Med* 1999;153:969.

U.S. Public Health Service. *Put prevention into practice: clinician's handbook of preventive services,* 2nd ed. International Medical Publishing, 1998:129.

Patient Resources/Education

Harvard School of Public Health. www.hsph.harvard.edu/headlice.html.

National Pediculosis Association. www.headlice.org.

7- to 9-Year Visit

HISTORY

As children age it becomes increasingly difficult to bring them to the office for well-child visits. Often well-child assessment can be incorporated into visits for illness or illness follow-up.

At this age many children are quite talkative. Ask about illnesses, accidents, or other concerns. How is the child doing in school? Is he receiving any special services? How are things in the home? Is the child brushing his teeth and wearing seat belts? Does he wear a bike helmet? Are there nutritional concerns? Any behaviors that cause concern?

PHYSICAL EXAMINATION

On physical examination, evaluate any areas of concern. In addition, examine:

Height/weight/blood pressure

Visual, auditory acuity

Heart

Abdomen

Signs of puberty

Signs of abuse

ANTICIPATORY GUIDANCE

Talking to your child

Family time

Limitation of TV

Positive reinforcement

Car safety—seat belts

Limitation of junk food

Escape from the house in case of fire

Appropriate protective equipment for sports

Learning to swim

Reminder about never swimming alone

Dangers of smoking

Children this age sleep 9 to 12 hours

Encouragement of physical fitness

Use of sun screens to decrease melanoma risk

HEALTH MAINTENANCE

Verify MMR, varicella, and hepatitis B immunization.

COMMON MEDICAL PROBLEMS

Herpes Labialis

Cold sores or recurrent gingivostomatitis are common during childhood. They usually occur during other illness or during psychologic stress. The infecting organism is typically herpes simplex virus type 1. Treatment consists of local application of petroleum jelly or systemic analgesics. Topical penciclovir 1% cream (Denavir) applied every 2 hours at the onset of pain and continued for 4 days has been shown to decrease the duration of pain from 4.1 days to 3.5 days. This medication should not be applied to mucous membranes and has not been studied in children. Topical acyclovir has not been shown to be effective. Oral acyclovir (Zovirax), 15 mg/kg five times daily for 7 days, is effective for primary gingivostomatitis. In immunocompromised hosts intravenous acyclovir prevents dissemination.

Patients should be advised that the lesion is contagious and can be spread to other areas of the body as well as to other people. In young children who mouth their toys, particular care should be taken to avoid sharing toys. Children with cold sores should not be restricted from school or day care. Newborns are susceptible to disseminated disease, so special precautions should be taken to avoid their exposure. Application of sunscreen, particularly in lip balm, may reduce recurrences due to sunlight exposure.

Growing Pains

Growing pains are defined as intermittent, aching pains in the thighs, calves, and back of the knees. They are seen in children and early adolescents and are not related to growing; however, they do tend to resolve with physical maturity. They are seen in approximately 2% of children. The pain usually occurs in the evening or night. Typically, the pain is bilateral, which distinguishes it from many, more serious causes of leg pain. This condition does not cause fever, limping, swelling, erythema, local tenderness, or limitations of range of motion. Evaluation consists of a thorough physical examination, with radiologic and other testing reserved for children with an atypical presentation. Treatment is supportive and includes analgesics such as acetaminophen, massage, or warm baths. Daily stretching exercises may help. Orthopedic referral should be considered if the symptoms worsen or if the diagnosis is in doubt.

REFERENCES

Abu-Arafeh I, Russell G. Recurrent limb pain in schoolchildren. *Arch Dis Child* 1996;74:336.

American Academy of Pediatrics. Herpes simplex. In: Peter G, ed. *1997 Red Book: report of the Committee on Infectious Diseases*, 24th ed. Elk Grove Village, IL: American Academy of Pediatrics, 1997:266.

Amir J, Harel L, Smetana Z, Varsano I. Treatment of herpes simplex gingivostomatitis with acyclovir in children: a randomised double blind placebo controlled study. *BMJ* 1997;314:1800.

Topical penciclovir for herpes labialis. *Med Lett* 1997;39:1003.

Nelson CT, Demmler GJ. Superficial HSV infection: How serious is it? What should you do? *Contemp Pediatr* 1996;13(5):96–111.

Peterson H. Growing pains. *Pediatr Clin North Am* 1986;33:1365.

10- to 12-Year Visit

HISTORY

The preadolescent may be very quiet in the office. Allow some time for private discussion with the child. Begin the conversation with topics of interest to the child. What do they do with friends? Do they play sports? Go to the mall? How is school going academically and socially? What is their diet like? Do they have any medical concerns? Do their friends use tobacco or drugs? Are their friends sexually active? Often adolescents answer sensitive questions about their friends sooner and more accurately than those about themselves. This allows the physician to ask about the patient. How is their sleep? What concerns does the parent have? Any illnesses or accidents?

PHYSICAL EXAMINATION

As the child matures, he may have great concern about being "normal." Reassure the child about normal aspects of the examination, especially the genital examination. Explain the examination and teach terms for body parts if this is necessary.

On examination pay particular attention to

Height/weight/blood pressure

Cardiovascular system

Musculoskeletal system

Signs of abuse

At this age, some authorities recommend the forward-bending test to evaluate for scoliosis. At present the U.S. Preventive Task Force finds insufficient evidence to recommend for or against screening. Sexual maturity ratings (Tanner staging) may also be done at this age (Table 2.19).

T ABLE 2.19. Sexual maturity rating (SMR, 10–12 years of age)

Boys

SMR Stage	Pubic Hair	Penis	Testes
1	None	Preadolescent size	Preadolescent size and appearance
2	Scanty, long, slightly pigmented	Slight enlargement	Enlarged scrotum, pink texture altered
3	Small amount, darker, starts to curl	Length increased	Larger
4	Resembles adult type, but less quantity; coarse, curly	Larger; glans and breadth increase in size	Larger, scrotum dark
5	Adult distribution, spread to medial surface of thighs	Adult size	Adult size

Girls

SMR Stage	Pubic Hair	Breasts
1	None	Preadolescent
2	Sparse amount at medial border of labia; lightly pigmented, straight	Breast and papilla elevated as small mound; areolar diameter increased
3	Increased amount, darker, beginning to curl	Breast and areola enlarged, no contour separation
4	Abundant, but less than in adult; coarse, curly	Areola and papilla form secondary mound
5	Adult feminine triangle, spread to medial surface of thighs	Mature; nipple projects, areola part of general breast contour

Reprinted from Behrman RE, ed. Nelson's textbook of pediatrics, 15th ed. Philadelphia: Saunders, 1996.

ANTICIPATORY GUIDANCE

As children mature sexually they have questions about whether they are normal. They may have difficulty coping with a new body image. Many parents have difficulty discussing these issues, and so children may obtain information, often incorrect, from friends. Parents should be encouraged to provide accurate information to their children. At this age many parents feel their children do not want them around. In reality, although they may not show it, most preadolescents want their parents' attention and greatly appreciate parental interest in their activities.

Other anticipatory guidance includes the following:

Talking to your child

Family meals

Limitation of TV

Positive reinforcement

Chores

Car safety

Limitation of junk food

HEALTH MAINTENANCE

Consider cholesterol screening if:

The family has a history of very high cholesterol.

There is premature coronary heart disease in a first-degree relative.

There are major nonlipid risk factors for coronary heart disease, such as smoking, hypertension, and diabetes.

Consider tuberculin skin testing if:

Children's parents (with unknown tuberculin skin test status) immigrated from regions of the world with a high prevalence of tuberculosis.

Children reside in areas with a high prevalence of tuberculosis (public health officials can identify high-risk neighborhoods or blocks).

Immunization—Td at age 10 and every year thereafter.

COMMON MEDICAL PROBLEMS

Scoliosis screening is controversial. One reason for this controversy is the lack of evidence that patients benefit from early detection. The possible risks of scoliosis include decreased pulmonary function and cosmetic effects. Use of an inexpensive scoliometer (Fig. 2.11) may decrease the need for radiologic evaluation. If scoliosis is detected, the child may be referred for a standing x-ray to measure the degree of curvature (Cobb angle). If the curvature is greater than 20° to 30° in the skeletally immature patient, orthopedic referral for possible bracing may be indicated. Surgery may be indicated for curves greater than 45°.

Menstrual concerns are common in young girls and their parents. Menstruation begins around age 13, earlier in African Americans. Evaluation is needed if there is no breast development by age 13 or no menarche by age 16. Cycles lasting greater than 8 to 10 days are considered abnormal. Many young girls have irregular menses secondary to anovulatory cycles. Girls should be taught to measure the length of the

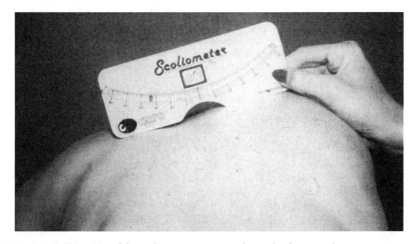

FIGURE 2.11. Use of the scoliometer to measure the angle of rotational prominence.

cycle from the onset of one cycle to the onset of the next. Many girls complain of dysmenorrhea. Because of their antiprogesterone effect, nonsteroidal antiinflammatory drugs can be very effective, especially if given the day before the anticipated onset of menses. Oral contraceptives may also alleviate the problem. Pregnancy must be ruled out whenever a girl has a prolonged interval between periods. Increased stress, exercise, or dieting may lead to anovulatory cycles.

REFERENCES

Well child care reference guide, 7th ed. Lexington, Kentucky: American Board of Family Practice, 1998.

Braverman PK, Sondheimer SJ. Menstrual disorders. *Pediatr Rev* 1997;18:17.

Scaggs DL. Adolescent idiopathic scoliosis: an update. *Am Fam Physician* 1996:53:2327.

U.S. Preventive Services Task Force. *Guide to clinical preventive services,* 2nd ed. Baltimore: Williams & Wilkins, 1996:517.

Adolescent Visits: Ages 13–15, 16–18, and 19–21

In the United States most adolescent health care is provided by family physicians. In many ways we are most suited to treat this age group, as we have experience dealing with child development as well as conditions such as gynecologic ones, more usually encountered in adults. In addition, we have the ability to treat the adolescent throughout the entire transition from childhood to adulthood, avoiding a change of providers. Despite these advantages, care of adolescents can be challenging. Teens may avoid eye contact and give one-word responses. Addressing issues of sexuality, substance abuse, and violence prevention is often troublesome. As family physicians we often have long-standing relationships with parents who may have difficulty with doctor/patient confidentiality between the physician and their child. Adolescents have the lowest rate of insurance coverage of any age group.

Yet adolescence is an exciting time of change, and as physicians we can help direct this change for the better. Most adolescent mortality is considered preventable, and we may be able to affect high-risk behaviors and unhealthy decisions favorably, although evidence of the effect of office intervention by the physician is not yet definitive.

The teen should be seen at least three times during adolescence, usually at ages 13 to 15, 16 to 18, and at 19 to 21. The emphasis of topics is varied with each visit so that all areas are addressed over time, and issues currently of particular importance are addressed at each visit.

CONFIDENTIALITY

Confidentiality issues in adolescence are often unique to this age group. In general, the patient's confidentiality should be respected unless the adolescent or someone else is at serious risk of harm. Confidentiality and consent statutes vary from state to state, so the physician should be aware of local laws. Usually, physicians discuss confidentiality during an office visit with parent and child present. Confidentiality may need to be reemphasized with the parent of the child, depending on the situation. The physician often encourages or offers to facilitate an open discussion with the parent. If the patient desires strict confidentiality, the adolescent may need to arrange payment personally to prevent parental notification by third-party payers.

HISTORY

History taking for adolescent visits can be facilitated by the use of a standardized form. Some teens are reluctant to speak at all or in the presence of a parent. Some time alone with the teen to discuss personal issues is essential. If the teen and the parent are interviewed together, speak to the teen first. Discussing nonthreatening issues such as after-school activities may open up conversation. Some teens require multiple visits before engaging in conversation easily. Ask about illnesses and nutrition. Are there menstrual concerns, such as pain or irregular periods? How is school going? Ask about friends and usual activities. Often asking about substance use or sexual activity in the friends before asking about them in the patient allows more open communication. Depending on the setting, the physician may need to prioritize the history and ask about issues presumed to be most important to this teen first, leaving other issues for a subsequent visit.

PHYSICAL EXAMINATION

During the physical examination reassure the teen about normal findings, especially of the genitalia. At this age teens are particularly conscious of their rapidly changing physical appearance. As many teens are concerned about contracting disease from the provider, attention to hand washing and cleanliness is especially important (Ginsburg).

On examination, areas of particular emphasis include the following:

Height, weight, blood pressure

Dentition

Lungs

Heart—murmurs

Abdomen

Skin for acne, evidence of abuse

External genitalia for hernia, testicular masses, and Tanner staging

Scoliosis screening

Pelvic examination if sexually active

DEVELOPMENT

Adolescents progress through the stages of early, middle, and late adolescence, although teens of the same age may be at different stages. Table 2.20 lists the developmental stages. Awareness of these may facilitate discussion with parents and teens.

ANTICIPATORY GUIDANCE — TEEN

As a group, adolescents are healthy. Leading causes of death are motor vehicle accidents, unintentional injury, homicide, and suicide. Therefore anticipatory guidance is usually the key element in the adolescent office visit. Unfortunately, many adolescents are reluctant to present for well visits, so prevention needs to be incorporated into visits for other purposes, such as acute illnesses, driver's physicals, or sports physicals. The HEADS mnemonic can facilitate recall of these important issues (Table 2.21). Some practices use a questionnaire completed by the patient to expedite and direct

T ABLE 2.20.   Developmental stages of adolescence

Stage	Age (Years)*	Tanner stage	Characteristics	Tasks

Early	11–14	I and II	Concern with body changes
			Egocentricity
			Ambivalence about
			   family relationships
				Separation from family
				Development of individual
				   identity and independence

Middle	14–17	III and IV	Concern with peer
			   group approval
			Increasing insistence on
			   control over decisions
			Increasing conflict with parents
			Feeling of invincibility
				Development of adult social
				   relationships with same
				   and opposite sex
				Continued struggle for identity
				   and independence

Late	17–22	V	Concern with life-planning issues
			Increasing commitment to
			   relationships
			Increasing ability to consider
			   consequences of own
			   behavior
				Development of career plans
				Development of moral/ethical
				   value system
				Maturation toward
				   autonomous
				   decision making

*The ages listed are guidelines; individuals go through these stages at different times.

From Alexander B, McGrew MC, Shore W. Adolescent sexuality issues in office practice. *Am Fam Physician* 1991;44:1273.

the office visit. Obviously, teens in different situations require emphasis of different aspects of anticipatory guidance.

SEXUALITY

Sexual concerns are frequent in adolescence, yet at times not voiced. Most adolescents benefit from reassurance of normality during the physical examination. Because not all patients are heterosexual, physicians should use care to not presume the gender of a patient's sexual partner. Gender-neutral phrases such as "dating" or "seeing anyone" may facilitate disclosure. Heterosexual and homosexual experimentation are common and may not predict future lifestyle choices. Adolescents may also be embarrassed if they are not sexually active. Abstinence should be encouraged. Many teens

T ABLE 2.21.   HEADS mnemonic for adolescent prevention

H—home, habits
E—education, employment, exercise
A—accidents, ambition, activities, abuse
D—drugs (tobacco, alcohol, others), diet, depression
S—sex, suicide

Adapted with permission from Goldenring JM, Cohen E. Getting into adolescent heads. *Contemp Pediatr* 1988; 5:75–90.

obtain most of their sexual education from friends, and so misinformation may need to be addressed. Similarly, physicians may need to teach a sexual vocabulary or learn local slang. Discussion of pregnancy prevention and prevention and recognition of sexually transmitted diseases may be appropriate.

ACCIDENT PREVENTION

As accidents are common causes of morbidity and mortality, discussion of their prevention is crucial. Common issues include the following:

Gun safety

Sports safety, including bicycle helmet use

Water safety

Consistent seat belt use

Avoidance of driving while impaired

Refusal of rides from impaired drivers

SUBSTANCE ABUSE

Most substance abuse begins in the teen years. Smokers should be encouraged to quit. Teens with alcohol or other substance abuse may need referral for rehabilitation. Many do not recognize the long-term consequences of current substance abuse. Some may be more likely to quit for an immediate small benefit than for a greater long-term benefit. For example, teen smokers may quit to avoid nicotine staining of their fingers or bad breath but not to prevent lung cancer.

DOMESTIC VIOLENCE

Teens may be in abusive relationships with parents, sexual partners, and peers. Many do not know where to receive assistance; therefore physicians should be aware of local resources. Cards for domestic violence centers placed in office restrooms are particularly effective since they can be accessed confidentially.

Other anticipatory guidance includes the following:

Use sunscreen; avoid excess sun exposure

See the dentist regularly

Exercise regularly

Avoid anabolic steroids, growth hormone

Consume 1,200–1,500 mg of calcium per day

Eat a low-fat, healthy diet

ANTICIPATORY GUIDANCE—PARENT

Parenting an adolescent can be challenging. Parents must change from being responsible for a child to interacting with another adult. The physician should explain the teen's development. Parents should be given the opportunity to express concerns about the teen and should be encouraged to monitor for signs of substance abuse such as substance use in friends, declining school or work performance, or rapid withdrawal from previous activities. Although teens may pretend to want to be left alone by their parents, most appreciate parental interest in their activities, including school activities or sports. Parents do well to learn about the teen's interests, even if these interests may not be their own. Positive reinforcement continues to be important. Teens should be encouraged but not forced to join after-school activities. An authoritative parenting style is generally more effective than an authoritarian or permissive one. The parent and teen should review the "house rules" periodically, with changes made as the child matures. Grounding or not allowing participation in activities or use of the phone can be effective punishments. Parents need to be consistent and firm with punishment.

HEALTH MAINTENANCE

Immunizations

Verify that the teen has received the hepatitis B series, Td, varicella vaccine (or the disease) and a second MMR. Chlamydia screening (usually at the time of the Pap smear) is recommended by the AAFP and others for asymptomatic sexually active adolescents. Pap smears are recommended by the AAFP for all sexually active women, at least every 3 years. Folic acid 0.4 mg/day (as found in most over-the-counter multivitamins) is recommended for women who are likely to become pregnant to prevent neural tube defects. Consider cholesterol screening in adolescents with a family history of very high cholesterol, premature coronary heart disease in a first-degree relative, or a personal risk factor for coronary heart disease. Tuberculosis screening is recommended for intravenous drug abusers, incarcerated or homeless youth, HIV-positive patients, those exposed to tuberculosis, and immigrants from countries with a high prevalence of tuberculosis. Although evidence of benefit is lacking, the physician may instruct the teen in self-examination of the breast or testicular examination.

COMMON MEDICAL PROBLEMS

Acne

Acne affects most teens at some point, usually beginning in early adolescence. Many affected teens suffer embarrassment and social stigmatization due to their appearance, though some fail to seek medical attention. Dietary restriction and topical cleansers are not effective and should be discouraged. Blackheads are open comedones whose color results from compacted follicular cells. They cannot be scrubbed away. In fact, aggressive cleansing can lead to increased inflammation. Acne is due to the overproduction of sebum, excessive desquamation of epithelial cells in the follicle, and secondary infection with *Propionibacterium acnes.* Treatment addresses these underlying causes and is determined by disease severity.

Comedonal acne presents in early adolescence with whiteheads and blackheads. *P. acnes* is not present at this stage. Treatment begins with topical tretinoin (Retin-A) (Table 2.22). Generally, creams are used; gels are reserved for very oily skin or very humid conditions. Therapy is started with the lowest concentration, two or three times weekly, and titrated up to daily use. If irritation develops, a lower concentration may be used or the medication may be applied less often. Sunscreens should be used consistently. Treatment usually requires several months. Once new lesions are no longer developing, the medication can be tapered.

Mild inflammatory acne presents with small papules and pustules. At this point colonization with *P. acnes* has occurred. Treatment consists of topical tretinoin combined with a topical antibiotic or benzoyl peroxide. As the condition resolves, the topical antibiotic may be tapered, followed by the tretinoin.

Inflammatory acne presents with comedones, papules, and pustules and at times deep, inflammatory nodules or cysts. Lesions occur on the face, trunk, and back. Treatment consists of an oral antibiotic effective against *P. acnes,* usually in combina-

TABLE 2.22. Topical medications used for acne

Medication	Formulation	Frequency	Comments
Tretinoin cream (Retin-A)	0.025%, 0.05%, 0.1%	Daily	Decrease concentration or use on alternate days if irritating May cause transient worsening May require 2–3 months for improvement
Tretinoin gel (Retin-A)	0.01% and 0.025%	Daily	Gel is more drying than cream Use sun screen Apply sparingly
Antibiotics			
Benzoyl peroxide gel (Benzac, Benzagel)	2.5%, 5%, 10%	Start every other day, titrate to twice daily over 2 weeks	2.5% as effective as higher concentrations Gels work best Can cause local irritation, allergic contact dermatitis—test on arm for a few hours before applying to face Aqueous base causes less drying than alcohol or acetone base Can bleach clothing
Erythromycin (Erycette, T-stat)	2% solution	Twice daily	Resistance becoming problematic
Clindamycin (Cleocin-T)	1% solution	Twice daily	Only 5% absorption Rarely causes pseudomembranous colitis
Erythromycin, 3% Benzoyl peroxide, 5% (Benzomycin)		Twice daily	Probably most effective topical antibiotic Decreased risk of antibiotic resistance with the combination

tion with topical tretinoin and a topical antibiotic. Choice of oral antibiotic depends on patient sensitivities, cost, and convenience. As the inflammation subsides, usually after 4 to 6 weeks, the oral antibiotic is discontinued and the topical medications are continued. As the condition resolves, these medications may be tapered as indicated earlier. If this treatment is ineffective, systemic treatment with isotretinoin (Accutane) may be needed, usually with specialist referral. This medication is highly effective but also highly teratogenic and may cause lipid abnormalities and musculoskeletal complaints. In women, resistant acne may be due to a hyperandrogenic state such as polycystic ovary syndrome. Treatment with oral contraceptives containing estrogen, especially with a less androgenic progestin, such as Desogen, Ortho-cept, or Ortho Tri-Cyclin, may be beneficial. If testosterone levels are elevated, treatment with spironolactone 100 to 200 mg/day can be effective.

Contraception

With the epidemic number of teen pregnancies in the United States, contraception is of the utmost importance. Teens are often misinformed about reproduction, do not plan intercourse, and therefore do not plan for contraception. Barrier and hormonal methods

TABLE **2.23.**   Contraception

Method	Percent of Women with Unintended Pregnancy in First Year of Use	Comments
Withdrawal	19	Commonly used by teens
Male condom	14	Protects against sexually transmitted diseases; see Table 2.3
Depo Provera	0.3	Many teens experience amenorrhea or irregular menses
Combined pill	3	Less than half of teens are still on the pill 1 year after prescription
		Teens should generally use a backup method for at least the first month of use, longer if there are frequent missed doses
		Many teens forget the pill, especially on weekends or when away from home
		Taking the pill at the same time each day may increase compliance
		Patients should be counseled on procedure if a pill is missed
		Backup is needed with concurrent use of seizure medications (barbiturates, dilantin, mysoline) and antibiotics (ampicillin, rifampicin, tetracycline)
No method	85%	

Adapted from U.S. Public Health Service. Put prevention into practice. In: *Clinician's handbook of preventive services,* 2nd ed. McLean, VA: International Medical Publishing, 1998.

can be quite effective if used correctly (Table 2.23). Yet many adolescents do not use their method correctly. In fact, many teens use withdrawal as their method of contraception. Contraceptive injections have the advantage of dosing every 3 months, but they do require office visits. Regardless of the method selected, frequent follow-up is necessary to verify that the teen is using the method and using it correctly.

PREVEN is the first emergency contraceptive pill approved in the United States. This kit contains a pregnancy test and four combined estrogen/progestin oral contraceptive pills. It is recommended for use within 72 hours of unprotected inter-

TABLE **2.24.**   Guidelines for proper condom use

Use latex rather than natural membrane condoms
Do not use torn or damaged condoms and avoid damaging them, as with teeth or fingernails
Put the condom on the penis before it touches the partner's genitals
Place the condom rim side up on the erect penis and unroll it to the base of the penis
Avoid air at the tip of the condom
Use a water-based lubricant such as KY Jelly or Astroglyde
Avoid oil-based lubricants such as petroleum jelly, cold cream, or mineral oil
Replace a broken condom immediately
After ejaculation hold the condom to the base of the erect penis before the penis is withdrawn

Adapted from the Centers for Disease Control and Prevention. 1998 Guidelines for the treatment of sexually transmitted diseases. *MMWR* 1998;47:1.

T ABLE 2.25. Treatment of sexually transmitted diseases (adolescent)

Disease	Treatment	Alternative	Comment
Primary and secondary syphilis	Benzathine penicillin G, 2.4 million units IM once	Doxycycline (Vibramycin), 100 mg twice daily for 2 weeks	Test also for HIV. Penicillin is the preferred choice
Genital herpes First episode	Acyclovir (Zovirax), 400 mg three times daily for 7–10 days	Valacyclovir (Valtrex), 1 g twice daily for 7–10 days	
Trichomonas	Metronidazole (Flagyl), 2 g orally once	Metronidazole, 500 mg twice daily for 7 days	Topical metronidazole is not not effective. Avoid concurrent use of alcohol
Chlamydia	Azithromycin (Zithromax), 1 g orally once	Doxycycline, 100 mg twice daily for 7 days	
Uncomplicated gonorrhea of cervix, urethra, or rectum	Ceftriaxone (Rocephin), 125 mg IM once	Cefixime (Suprax), 400 mg orally once	Treat for Chlamydia concurrently

Adapted from Centers for Disease Control and Prevention. 1998 Guidelines for the Treatment of Sexually Transmitted Diseases. *MMWR* 1998;47:1.

course, with probable higher efficacy if used in the first 24 hours. The pregnancy rate from a single act of intercourse is reduced from 8/100 to 2/100 (PREVEN package insert). Once this is prescribed, the physician has an opportunity to assist the patient with longer-term contraception.

Sexually Transmitted Diseases

Sexually active adolescents are highly prone to sexually transmitted diseases. After abstinence, condoms are the most effective method to prevent infection. To be effective, condoms need to be available at the time of sexual activity and the teen needs to be educated on their use (Table 2.24). The CDC has recently updated its recommendations on the treatment of sexually transmitted diseases (Table 2.25). Treatment of partners is also necessary.

REFERENCES

Alexander B, McGrew MC, Shore W. Adolescent sexuality issues in office practice. *Am Fam Physician* 1991;44:1273.

Centers for Disease Control and Prevention. 1998 guidelines for the treatment of sexually transmitted diseases. *MMWR* 1998;47:1.

Gilchrist V, Alexander E. Preventive health care for adolescents. *Prim Care* 1994;21:759.

Ginsburg KR, et al. Adolescents' perceptions of factors affecting their decisions to seek health care. *JAMA* 1995;273:1913.

Leyden JJ. Drug therapy for acne vulgaris. *N Engl J Med* 1997;336:1156.

Montalto NJ. Implementing the guidelines for adolescent preventive services. *Am Fam Physician* 1998;57:2181.

Strasburger VC. Acne: what every pediatrician needs to know. *Pediatr Clin North Am* 1997;44:1505.

Preparticipation Examination

Family physicians are frequently called on to evaluate children and adolescents before athletic participation. These examinations may occur in the office or may be done for a large group of students in the school. In any case, the physician must do an efficient, thorough evaluation. This section will focus on the screening evaluation. Ideally, the preparticipation examination should occur 6 weeks before the start of practice, to allow time for supplemental evaluation before practice starts.

HISTORY

The history will uncover most of the abnormalities detected on a screening evaluation. Unfortunately, most adolescents cannot accurately recall their medical history. The best way to obtain the history is with a questionnaire, completed by the child and parent together before the examination. Figure 2.12 is the form endorsed by the AAFP. At the time of the examination the physician should review the information, paying particular attention to the abnormalities noted and any cardiovascular or orthopedic complaints.

PHYSICAL EXAMINATION

The physical examination concentrates on areas of greatest concern with sports participation, usually the cardiovascular and musculoskeletal systems. To some degree the examination is individualized for the particular sport (e.g., more emphasis on the knee examination for football than for golf).

Table 2.26 outlines the components of the preparticipation physical examination, and Table 2.27 demonstrates the general screening musculoskeletal examination. If an abnormality is detected, a more detailed examination of that area is indicated.

LABORATORY EVALUATION

Routine laboratory testing in the asymptomatic athlete is unnecessary. Similarly, electrocardiograms, echocardiography, exercise stress testing, and spirometry are not routinely indicated. Supplemental testing may be needed based on the history and physical examination.

CLEARANCE

If the evaluation is normal the athlete is cleared for participation. If the evaluation is abnormal, clearance becomes more difficult. If the evaluation is abnormal in a mass

Preparticipation Physical Evaluation

HISTORY

DATE OF EXAM _____

Name _____ Sex _____ Age _____ Date of birth _____

Grade ____ School _____ Sport(s) _____

Address _____ Phone _____

Personal physician _____

In case of emergency, contact

Name _____ Relationship _____ Phone (H) _____ (W) _____

Explain "Yes" answers below.
Circle questions you don't know the answers to.

Yes No

1. Have you had a medical illness or injury since your last check up or sports physical? ☐ ☐
   Do you have an ongoing or chronic illness? ☐ ☐
2. Have you ever been hospitalized overnight? ☐ ☐
   Have you ever had surgery? ☐ ☐
3. Are you currently taking any prescription or nonprescription (over-the-counter) medications or pills or using an inhaler? ☐ ☐
   Have you ever taken any supplements or vitamins to help you gain or lose weight or improve your performance? ☐ ☐
4. Do you have any allergies (for example, to pollen, medicine, food, or stinging insects)? ☐ ☐
   Have you ever had a rash or hives develop during or after exercise? ☐ ☐
5. Have you ever passed out during or after exercise? ☐ ☐
   Have you ever been dizzy during or after exercise? ☐ ☐
   Have you ever had chest pain during or after exercise? ☐ ☐
   Do you get tired more quickly than your friends do during exercise? ☐ ☐
   Have you ever had racing of your heart or skipped heartbeats? ☐ ☐
   Have you had high blood pressure or high cholesterol? ☐ ☐
   Have you ever been told you have a heart murmur? ☐ ☐
   Has any family member or relative died of heart problems or of sudden death before age 50? ☐ ☐
   Have you had a severe viral infection (for example, myocarditis or mononucleosis) within the last month? ☐ ☐
   Has a physician ever denied or restricted your participation in sports for any heart problems? ☐ ☐
6. Do you have any current skin problems (for example, itching, rashes, acne, warts, fungus, or blisters)? ☐ ☐
7. Have you ever had a head injury or concussion? ☐ ☐
   Have you ever been knocked out, become unconscious, or lost your memory? ☐ ☐
   Have you ever had a seizure? ☐ ☐
   Do you have frequent or severe headaches? ☐ ☐
   Have you ever had numbness or tingling in your arms, hands, legs, or feet? ☐ ☐
   Have you ever had a stinger, burner, or pinched nerve? ☐ ☐
8. Have you ever become ill from exercising in the heat? ☐ ☐
9. Do you cough, wheeze, or have trouble breathing during or after activity? ☐ ☐
   Do you have asthma? ☐ ☐
   Do you have seasonal allergies that require medical treatment? ☐ ☐

Yes No

10. Do you use any special protective or corrective equipment or devices that aren't usually used for your sport or position (for example, knee brace, special neck roll, foot orthotics, retainer on your teeth, hearing aid)? ☐ ☐
11. Have you had any problems with your eyes or vision? ☐ ☐
    Do you wear glasses, contacts, or protective eyewear? ☐ ☐
12. Have you ever had a sprain, strain, or swelling after injury? ☐ ☐
    Have you broken or fractured any bones or dislocated any joints? ☐ ☐
    Have you had any other problems with pain or swelling in muscles, tendons, bones, or joints? ☐ ☐
    If yes, check appropriate box and explain below.
    ☐ Head   ☐ Elbow   ☐ Hip
    ☐ Neck   ☐ Forearm   ☐ Thigh
    ☐ Back   ☐ Wrist   ☐ Knee
    ☐ Chest   ☐ Hand   ☐ Shin/calf
    ☐ Shoulder   ☐ Finger   ☐ Ankle
    ☐ Upper arm   ☐ Foot
13. Do you want to weigh more or less than you do now? ☐ ☐
    Do you lose weight regularly to meet weight requirements for your sport? ☐ ☐
14. Do you feel stressed out? ☐ ☐
15. Record the dates of your most recent immunizations (shots) for:
    Tetanus _____ Measles _____
    Hepatitis B _____ Chickenpox _____

FEMALES ONLY

16. When was your first menstrual period? _____
    When was your most recent menstrual period? _____
    How much time do you usually have from the start of one period to the start of another? _____
    How many periods have you had in the last year? _____
    What was the longest time between periods in the last year? _____

Explain "Yes" answers here: _____
_____
_____
_____
_____
_____
_____
_____
_____

I hereby state that, to the best of my knowledge, my answers to the above questions are complete and correct.

Signature of athlete _____ Signature of parent/guardian _____ Date _____

FIGURE 2.12. Preparticipation physical evaluation form. From Preparticipation Physical Evaluation, 2nd ed. New York: McGraw Hill, 1997. Reprinted by permission, American Academy of Family Physicians, American Academy of Pediatrics, American Medical Society for Sports Medicine, American Occupaedic Society for Sports Medicine, and American Osteopathic Academy of Sports Medicine.

T ABLE 2.26.   Standard components of the preparticipation physical examination

Height	Genitalia (males only)
Weight	Single or undescended testicle
Eyes	Testicular mass
Visual acuity (Snellen chart)	Hernia
Differences in pupil size	Skin
Oral cavity	Rashes
Ears	Lesions
Nose	Musculoskeletal system
Lungs	Contour range of motion stability and symmetry of
Cardiovascular system	neck, back, shoulder/arm, elbow/forearm,
Blood pressure	wrist/hand, hip/thigh, knee, leg/ankle, foot
Pulses (radial, femoral)	
Heart (rate, rhythm, murmurs)	
Abdomen	
Masses	
Tenderness	
Organomegaly	

From Preparticipation Physical Evaluation, 2nd ed. New York: McGraw Hill, 1997. Reprinted by permission, American Academy of Family Physicians, American Academy of Pediatrics, American Medical Society for Sports Medicine, American Occupaedic Society for Sports Medicine, and American Osteopathic Academy of Sports Medicine.

screening evaluation, in most cases the athlete is referred to the primary physician or a specialist for further evaluation. Table 2.28 lists common medical condition and recommendations for sports participation. Table 2.29 lists common concerns related to some common sports.

Medical/Legal Considerations

If a physician advises restricted participation, an athlete may have the right to participate against medical advice. The athlete may seek a second medical opinion. Many experts recommend that the athlete and parents, if the athlete is a minor, sign a waiver. This document outlines the medical concerns regarding participation and releases the physician and sponsoring organization from liability. Specialty consultation and legal counsel may be needed.

REFERENCES

Preparticipation physical evaluation, 2nd ed. New York: McGraw-Hill 1997.

Roberts WO. Certifying wrestler's minimum weight: a new requirement. *Phys Sports Med* 1998;26: 79–81.

Rome ES. Sports-related Injuries among adolescents: When do they occur and how can we prevent them? *Pediatr Rev* 1995:16:184.

TABLE 2.27. The "2-minute" orthopedic examination

Instruction and Maneuvers	Possible Abnormalities to Observe
Stand facing examiner	Enlarged or prominent acromioclavicular joint (acromioclavicular sprain)
	Enlarged or prominent sternoclavicular joint (sternoclavicular sprain)
	Asymmetry of hips (due to scoliosis or leg length discrepancy)
	Swollen knee
	Swollen ankle
Look at the ceiling (floor)	Decreased range of motion suggesting prior injury or congenital abnormality
Touch your right (left) ear to your right (left) shoulder	
Turn your head to the right (left)	
Shrug your shoulders (examiner resists)	Trapezius weakness
Hold your arms out to your sides (examiner resists)	Deltoid weakness
Place your hands behind your head (shoulder abduction and external rotation)	Decreased range of motion suggesting prior shoulder injury (e.g., rotator cuff tendinitis or tear, subluxation or dislocation, acromioclavicular sprain)
Place your hands behind your back (shoulder adduction and internal rotation)	
Bend and straighten your elbows	Decreased range of motion
With your arms at your sides and your elbows bent, turn your hands over	Decreased pronation or supination
Spread your fingers, make a fist	Decreased range of motion or deformity
Tighten your thigh muscles	Asymmetry of muscle bulk or knee swelling suggesting prior knee injury
Stand on your heels	Decreased strength of muscles of anterior leg and ankle sprain
Turn around (stand with back to examiner)	Shoulder asymmetry, pelvic tilt (due to leg length discrepancy)
Stand on your toes	Decreased strength or bulk of muscles of posterior leg (calf)
With your knees straight, bend forward and touch your toes	Decreased hamstring flexibility, scoliosis
Walking like a duck, take four steps	Inability to complete maneuver with buttocks on heels suggests prior knee or ankle injury

From Dershewitz RA, ed. Ambulatory pediatric care, 3rd ed. New York: Lippincott Williams & Wilkins, 1998. Reprinted by permission.

T ABLE 2.28. Medical conditions and sports participation

This table is designed to be understood by medical and nonmedical personnel. In the "Explanation" section below, "needs evaluation" means that a physician with appropriate knowledge and experience should assess the safety of a given sport for an athlete with the listed medical condition. Unless otherwise noted, this is because of the variability of the severity of the disease or of the risk of injury among the specific sports, or both.

Condition	May Participate
Atlantoaxial instability (instability of the joint between cervical vertebrae 1 and 2)	Qualified Yes
Explanation: Athlete needs evaluation to assess risk of spinal cord injury during sports participation.	
Bleeding disorder	Qualified Yes
Explanation: Athlete needs evaluation.	
Cardiovascular diseases	
Carditis (inflammation of the heart)	No
Explanation: Carditis may result in sudden death with exertion.	
Hypertension (high blood pressure)	Qualified Yes
Explanation: Those with significant essential (unexplained) hypertension should avoid weight and power lifting, body building, and strength training. Those with secondary hypertension (hypertension caused by a previously identified disease), or severe essential hypertension, need evaluation.	
Congenital heart disease (structural heart defects present at birth)	Qualified Yes
Explanation: Those with mild forms may participate fully; those with moderate or severe forms, or who have undergone surgery, need evaluation.	
Dysrhythmia (irregular heart rhythm)	Qualified Yes
Explanation: Athlete needs evaluation because some types require therapy or make certain sports dangerous, or both.	
Mitral valve prolapse (abnormal heart valve)	Qualified Yes
Explanation: Those with symptoms (chest pain, symptoms of possible dysrhythmia) or evidence of mitral regurgitation (leaking) on physical examination need evaluation. All others may participate fully.	
Heart murmur	Qualified Yes
Explanation: If the murmur is innocent (does not indicate heart disease), full participation is permitted. Otherwise, the athlete needs evaluation (see "Congenital heart disease" and "Mitral valve prolapse" above).	

Cerebral palsy	Qualified Yes
Explanation: Athlete needs evaluation.	
Diabetes mellitus	Yes
Explanation: All sports can be played with proper attention to diet, hydration, and insulin therapy. Particular attention is needed for activities that last 30 minutes or more.	
Diarrhea	Qualified No
Explanation: Unless disease is mild, no participation is permitted, because diarrhea may increase the risk of dehydration and heat illness. See "Fever" below.	
Eating disorders	
Anorexia nervosa, Bulimia nervosa	Qualified Yes
Explanation: These patients need both medical and psychiatric assessment before participation.	
Eyes	
Functionally one-eyed athlete, loss of an eye, detached retina, previous eye surgery or serious eye injury	Qualified Yes
Explanation: A functionally one-eyed athlete has a best corrected visual acuity of <20/40 in the worse eye. These athletes would suffer significant disability if the better eye was seriously injured as would those with loss of an eye. Some athletes who have previously undergone eye surgery or had a serious eye injury may have an increased risk of injury because of weakened eye tissue. Availability of eye guards approved by the American Society for Testing Materials (ASTM) and other protective equipment may allow participation in most sports, but this must be judged on an individual basis.	
Fever	No
Explanation: Fever can increase cardiopulmonary effort, reduce maximum exercise capacity, make heat illness more likely, and increase orthostatic hypotension during exercise. Fever may rarely accompany myocarditis or other infections that may make exercise dangerous.	
Heat illness, history of	Qualified Yes
Explanation: Because of the increase likelihood of recurrence, the athlete needs individual assessment to determine the presence of predisposing conditions and to arrange a prevention strategy.	
HIV infection	Yes
Explanation: Because of the apparent minimal risk to others, all sports may be played that the state of health allows. In all athletes, skin lesions should be properly covered, and athletic personnel should use universal precautions when handling blood or body fluids with visible blood.	

continued

TABLE 2.28. Medical conditions and sports participation (continued)

Condition	May Participate
Kidney: absence of one	Qualified Yes
Explanation: Athlete needs individual assessment for contact/collision and limited contact sports.	
Liver, enlarged	Qualified Yes
Explanation: If the liver is acutely enlarged, participation should be avoided because of risk of rupture. If the liver is chronically enlarged, individual assessment is needed before contact/collision or limited contact sports are played.	
Malignancy	Qualified Yes
Explanation: Athlete needs individual assessment.	
Musculoskeletal disorders	Qualified Yes
Explanation: Athlete needs individual assessment.	
Neurologic	
History of serious head or spine trauma, severe or repeated concussions, or craniotomy	Qualified Yes
Explanation: Athlete needs individual assessment for contact/collision or limited contact sports, and also for noncontact sports if there are deficits in judgment or cognition. Recent research supports a conservative approach to management of concussion.	
Convulsive disorder, well controlled	Yes
Explanation: Risk of convulsion during participation is minimal.	
Convulsive disorder, poorly controlled	Qualified Yes
Explanation: Athlete needs individual assessment for contact/collision or limited contact sports. Avoid the following noncontact sports: archery, riflery, swimming, weight or power lifting, strength training, or sports involving heights. In these sports, occurrence of a convulsion may be a risk to self or others.	
Obesity	Qualified Yes
Explanation: Because of the risk of heat illness, obese persons need careful acclimatization and hydration.	
Organ transplant recipient	Qualified Yes
Explanation: Athlete needs individual assessment.	
Ovary: absence of one	Yes
Explanation: Risk of severe injury to the remaining ovary is minimal.	

Respiratory

Pulmonary compromise including cystic fibrosis — Qualified Yes

Explanation: Athlete needs individual assessment, but generally all sports may be played if oxygenation remains satisfactory during a graded exercise test. Patients with cystic fibrosis need acclimatization and good hydration to reduce the risk of heat illness.

Asthma — Yes

Explanation: With proper medication and education, only athletes with the most severe asthma will have to modify their participation.

Acute upper respiratory infection — Qualified Yes

Explanation: Upper respiratory obstruction may affect pulmonary function. Athlete needs individual assessment for all but mild disease. See "Fever" above.

Sickle cell disease — Qualified Yes

Explanation: Athlete needs individual assessment. In general, if status of the illness permits, all but high-exertion, contact/collision sports may be played. Overheating, dehydration, and chilling must be avoided.

Sickle cell trait — Yes

Explanation: It is unlikely that individuals with sickle cell trait (AS) have an increased risk of sudden death or other medical problems during athletic participation except under the most extreme conditions of heat, humidity, and possibly increased altitude. These individuals, like all athletes, should be carefully conditioned, acclimatized, and hydrated to reduce any possible risk.

Skin: boils, herpes simplex, impetigo, scabies, molluscum contagiosum — Qualified Yes

Explanation: While the patient is contagious, participation in gymnastics with mats, martial arts, wrestling, or other contact/collision or limited contact sports is not allowed. Herpes simplex virus probably is not transmitted via mats.

Spleen, enlarged — Qualified Yes

Explanation: Patient with acutely enlarged spleens should avoid all sports because of risk of rupture. Those with chronically enlarged spleens need individual assessment before playing contact/collision or limited contact sports.

Testicle: absent or undescended — Yes

Explanation: Certain sports may require a protective cup.

Adapted with permission from: American Academy of Pediatrics Committee on Sports Medicine and Fitness: Medical conditions affecting sports participation. Pediatrics 1994;94(5):757–760.

T ABLE 2.29. Common sport specific concerns

Baseball	Leading cause of sports-related eye injury; batting helmets should have shatter-resistant face shields
Football	"Spearing" (using the head for blocking) increases spine injuries; adequate fluids must be available at games and practices
Gymnastics	High risk for eating disorders; prone to amenorrhea
Wrestling	Showering and mat scrubbing can reduce the risk of infectious disease; dehydration and dieting to "make weight" can be lethal
	Calculating a wrestler's minimum weight requires an estimation of body fat using high-precision calipers (see Roberts 1998).

CHAPTER 3

Infectious Diseases

Fever of Unknown Origin

CHIEF COMPLAINT

"My child has a fever."

HISTORY OF PRESENT ILLNESS

Fever is a very common complaint in the pediatric age group. The family physician's task is to differentiate the very few children with fever and severe illness from the very many children with fever and uncomplicated viral illness. The history must include the duration of illness and the presence of seizures, confusion, wheezing, cough, vomiting, diarrhea, dysuria, rash, and joint or dental pain. The method of taking the temperature, recent antipyretics, and whether the child was overbundled are particularly important if the child is less febrile in the office than at home. In general, axillary, tympanic, and temperatures taken with adhesive strips or pacifier thermometers may underestimate fever but rarely overestimate it. A history of recent hospitalization, immunizations, exposure to infectious diseases as well as recent use of antibiotics or other medications should be explored.

MEDICAL HISTORY

Most chronic medical problems can predispose a child to serious complications from infectious disease. For example, fever in the child with immunosuppression or oncologic disease is often serious and requires individualized management. Birth history—including prematurity, perinatal antibiotic use, and neonatal complications—is particularly important in infants. The clinician should verify that the immunizations, especially that for *Haemophilus* influenza, are up to date.

SOCIAL HISTORY

Much of the home management of the child with fever relies on close observation of the child by competent caregivers. Assessment of the reliability of the caregivers, as well as access to transportation and a telephone, is essential.

PHYSICAL EXAMINATION

The physical examination begins with an accurate measurement of the temperature. The rectal temperature is most reliable. A normal temperature on axillary or tympanic measurement does not exclude the possibility of fever. The most reliable predictor of serious etiology of fever is toxic appearance of the child. This appearance includes irritability, decreased attentiveness, poor feeding, poor eye contact, decreased socialization, decreased playfulness, poor perfusion, cyanosis, and lethargy. Obviously, toxic appearance is more easily assessed in older children than in young infants. The remainder of

85

the examination assesses the child for focal signs of infection. These include ocular discharge, otitis media, cough, wheezes or rhonchi, nuchal rigidity, abdominal tenderness, arthritis, rash, and cellulitis. Adenopathy may guide the clinician to a source of infection.

MANAGEMENT

Management of the febrile child varies with the clinical presentation and age of the child. When a source for the fever is found, the fever is controlled by managing the underlying condition. When a child appears toxic, hospitalization and a septic workup are indicated. In the child who is less than 1 month of age, hospitalization and full septic workup—including culture of cerebrospinal fluid (CSF), blood, and urine, and if diarrhea is present, evaluation of stool for white blood cells—are usually recommended. In infants 1 to 3 months of age, assessment of "toxic" appearance is still less reliable than that in older children, and so most authorities recommend urinalysis, complete blood cell count (CBC), and cultures of blood and urine. The white blood cell count (WBC) should not be used to decide whether to do a lumbar puncture, as the WBC is often lower in children with meningitis than in those with occult bacteremia. If the child meets low-risk criteria (Table 3.1), he or she may be managed as an outpatient. If CSF has been obtained, empiric treatment with a dose of ceftriaxone (Rocephin) 50 mg/kg may be given. If CSF has not been obtained, empiric use of antibiotics is discouraged, as an underlying meningitis may be masked.

Management of fevers without an underlying source in children older than 3 months has long been controversial. Fevers are commonly caused by viral illnesses and require only supportive treatment. However, some fevers are caused by underlying bacteremia, which may occasionally lead to sepsis or meningitis. The goal is to identify the few children at risk for severe complications while subjecting as few children as possible to invasive testing. The risk of bacteremia increases with increasing temperature, yet even with a temperature of 106° Fahrenheit only 26% of children are bacteremic. Guidelines have been written that recommend obtaining blood cultures and using the WBC to decide whether to use empiric ceftriaxone. This approach is difficult to implement in most offices and may not lead to improved outcome. In the office setting, the most reasonable approach is to evaluate the home setting. If the caregivers are competent, they should observe the child closely. If the child's condition deteriorates, which includes increased lethargy, decreased appetite, or focal complaints, the child should be rechecked. If the fever persists for 2 more days, the child

TABLE 3.1. Low-risk criteria for infants 1–3 months of age with fever

Previously healthy
Well appearance
No focal bacterial infection on examination, except otitis media
WBC 5,000–15,000/mm^3
<1,500 bands/mm^3
Normal urinalysis
When diarrhea present, <5 WBC/high power field
Reliable social situation

Abbreviation: WBC, white blood cell count.

Adapted from Jaskiewicz JA. Febrile Infants at Low Risk for Serious Bacterial Infection—An Appraisal of the Rochester Criteria and Implication for Management. *Pediatrics* 1994;94:390; and Baraff LJ, et al. Practice guideline for the management of infants and children 0 to 36 months of age with fever without source. *Pediatrics* 1993;92:1.

should be rechecked. If the caregivers are believed to be unreliable, daily examinations or a blood culture may improve surveillance of the child. Empiric antibiotics are usually not needed.

Supportive treatment with antipyretics can be considered, but only for the child's comfort. In general, acetaminophen should be used first; ibuprofen can be used if this is ineffective (see Table A.3 in the Appendix).

If the fever persists more than 2 days, the physical examination should be repeated, again looking for focal signs of infection. At this point urine culture should be obtained in girls less than 2 years of age, boys less than 6 months of age, or any child with urinary symptoms. In a child off antibiotics, a negative culture on urine culture from a bagged specimen rules out a urinary tract infection. If the culture is positive from a bagged specimen, it may be a contaminant (see Chapter 6).

Many conditions—including infections, connective tissue disorders, and malignancies—may present with persistent fever. Children with persistent fevers require individualized evaluation and management, which is described elsewhere. Because Kawasaki's disease and rheumatic fever have been shown to improve with directed treatment, these conditions should not be overlooked.

PATIENT EDUCATION

Parents are concerned when their child has fever, yet fever itself is rarely harmful and may play a beneficial role in the eradication of infection. Antipyretics are used mainly for the comfort of the child. Because of the risk of Reyes syndrome, aspirin should not be used for fever in children. Sponge baths are usually unnecessary and are uncomfortable for the child. Extra fluids can be encouraged but not forced.

REFERENCES

American Academy of Pediatrics. Kawasaki disease. In: Peter G, ed. *1997 Red Book: report of the Committee on Infectious Diseases*, 24th ed. Elk Grove Village, IL: American Academy of Pediatrics, 1997:316.

Avner JR. Occult bacteremia: How great the risk? *Contemp Pediatr* 1997;14:53.

Baraff LJ, et al. Practice guideline for the management of infants and children 0 to 36 months of age with fever without source. *Pediatrics* 1993;92:1.

Bonandio WA. The history and physical assessments of the febrile infant. *Pediatr Clin North Am* 1998;45:65.

Jaskiewicz JA, et al. Febrile infants at low risk for serious bacterial infection: an appraisal of the Rochester criteria and implication for management. *Pediatrics* 1994;94:390.

Kramer MS, Shapiro ED. Management of the young febrile child: a commentary on the recent practice guidelines. *Pediatrics* 1997;100:128.

Lopez JA, et al. Managing fever in infants and toddlers: toward a standard of care. *Postgrad Med* 1997;101:241.

McCarthy PL, et al. Fever without apparent source on clinical examination, and lower respiratory infections in children, other infectious diseases, and acute gastroenteritis in early childhood. *Curr Opin Pediatr* 1997;9:105.

McCarthy PL, et al. Fever without apparent source on clinical examination, infectious diseases, and lower respiratory infections in children. *Curr Opin Pediatr* 1998;10:101.

Schmidt B. *Your child's health.* New York: Bantam, 1991.

Otitis Media

Otitis media is divided into two distinct entities, acute otitis media and otitis media with effusion. **Acute otitis media** is defined as the presence of fluid in the middle ear in association with signs or symptoms of acute local or systemic illness, such as otalgia, otorrhea, bulging red or bulging yellow tympanic membrane, and fever. **Otitis media with effusion** is defined as fluid in the middle ear without signs or symptoms of acute infection.

CHIEF COMPLAINT

"My ear hurts.""My child has a fever and is tugging at his ear."

HISTORY

Ear pain is present in 47% to 83% of children with acute otitis media. Conversely, otalgia may be seen in children who do not have acute otitis media. In one study, half the children with ear pain did not have acute otitis media. Another study found that only 12% of children "pulling at the ear" had acute otitis media. Fever is also frequently present, but it is usually low grade and lasts less than 24 hours. Nearly all children with acute otitis media have either cough or rhinitis. According to Weiss, in the setting of an upper respiratory infection, otalgia predicted acute otitis media 83% of the time.

Acute otitis media is more common in children who are bottlefed, attend day care, and are between the ages of 6 and 18 months.

Otitis media with effusion may be an incidental finding in an otherwise well child or may be seen in a child with an acute illness. Some children present with a sensation of popping or fluid in the ear.

PHYSICAL EXAMINATION

Appropriate equipment is necessary for the accurate diagnosis of otitis media. For optimal visualization the light source must emit 100 foot-candles, which requires replacing the otoscope bulb after every 20 hours of use. Cerumen occluding more than 25% of the tympanic membrane should be removed with either a plastic loop or a spoon. Parents should be warned before the start of removal that there is a slight risk of bleeding. In the office, triethanolamine polypeptide (Cerumenex) may be placed in the ear 15 to 30 minutes before warm-water lavage to allow for easier removal. In preparation for an office visit, glycerine or carbamide peroxide (Debrox) can be used at home twice a day for up to 4 days.

FIGURE 3.1. **A:** Normal tympanometric pattern. The compliance curve is peaked (indicating normal mobility of the tympanic membrane), and the peak occurs at a pressure of -10 mm H_2O (normal pressure: $+100$ mm H_2O to -150 mm H_2O). The ear canal volume is normal (normal volume: 0.2 mL to 2.0 mL). **B:** Flat tympanometric pattern typical of fluid within the middle ear. The ear volume is normal, whereas mobility is greatly reduced. This pattern is also seen with scarred, sclerotic tympanic membranes. In actual clinical practice, tympanograms are rarely absolutely flat, but usually show some evidence of minimal mobility. **C:** The compliance curve appears normal, but the peak occurs at -200 mm H_2O, indicating an abnormal pressure within the middle ear. This pattern is characteristic of a blocked eustachian tube.

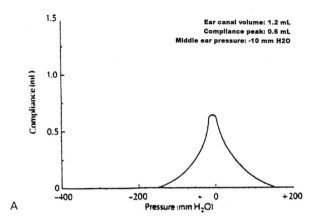

Ear canal volume: 1.2 mL
Compliance peak: 0.6 mL
Middle ear pressure: -10 mm H2O

A

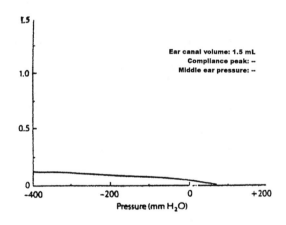

Ear canal volume: 1.5 mL
Compliance peak: --
Middle ear pressure: --

B

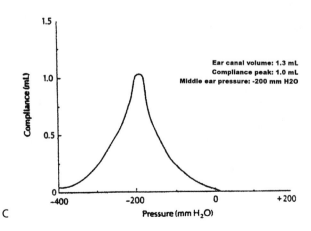

Ear canal volume: 1.3 mL
Compliance peak: 1.0 mL
Middle ear pressure: -200 mm H2O

C

Pneumatic otoscopy allows the detection of an effusion, as fluid behind the tympanic membrane decreases mobility. Pneumatic otoscopy requires an airtight system, which is achieved more easily with a rubber-tipped ear speculum, and practice. Excessive pressure must be avoided or the drum will move even in the presence of an effusion. Bulging, cloudy, and distinctly red tympanic membranes in the presence of an effusion are indicative of acute otitis media. Unfortunately, all these findings may be present to a greater or lesser degree, thus complicating the diagnosis of acute otitis media. The mastoid should be palpated for tenderness. The remainder of the exam excludes concurrent illness

Tympanometry records the compliance of the middle ear as air pressure is increased in the external canal. This compliance decreases in the presence of an effusion. Tympanometry can facilitate the detection of an effusion and is especially helpful when pneumatic otoscopy is inconclusive. Figure 3.1 depicts tympanograms of the normal ear and the ear with an effusion.

In otitis media with effusion, a middle ear effusion is present, with no other changes of the tympanic membrane, and without symptoms of acute infection.

MANAGEMENT OF ACUTE OTITIS MEDIA

Currently, the approach to the management of **acute otitis media** is undergoing a transformation. Eighty percent of acute otitis media cases resolve without antibiotics. Most children will be pain-free at 24 hours without antibiotics, but the use of antibiotics has been shown to decrease the pain severity. With the increasing frequency of antibiotic resistance, antibiotics should be reserved for definite acute otitis media. When the diagnosis is not certain, follow-up of the child without antibiotic therapy is recommended. Table 3.2 lists antibiotics commonly prescribed for otitis media. Amoxicillin (Amoxil) remains the antibiotic of first choice since it is economical and effective. With the increasing incidence of pneumococcal resistance to penicillin, some experts are recommending that high-dose amoxicillin (80 to 90 mg/kg/day) be used for initial empiric therapy. Ideally, the need for the increased dose depends on the local prevalence, but this information may not be readily available to the clinicians (Dowell, 1999). Short-course therapy of 5 to 7 days is recommended for children beyond the age of 2 years with none of the following:

Perforation of the tympanic membrane

Chronic or recurrent acute otitis media

Craniofacial abnormalities

Immunocompromised condition.

Other children should receive 10 to 14 days of therapy. Topical anesthetic drops (Auralgan) provide symptomatic relief, either with or without antibiotics. A single dose of intramuscular ceftriaxone (Rocephin) (50 mg/kg) is as effective as a 10-day course of amoxicillin or trimethoprim sulfamethoxazole (Bactrim) for penicillin-sensitive pneumococcus. This option may be particularly useful for recurrent cases, noncompliant patients, or cases in which antibiotics have failed. If penicillin-resistant pneumococcus is suspected as the cause of antibiotic failure, a 3-day course of intramuscular ceftriaxone (50 mg/kg/day) or high-dose amoxicillin with clavulanate (Augmentin) may be effective.

FOLLOW-UP

The child should be seen again if symptoms increase despite treatment or if they persist beyond the first 2 to 4 days after treatment. At this point, a second-line antibiotic may be used. If the second antibiotic fails, a third-line antibiotic should be used. If this

T ABLE 3.2.   Recommended drugs for medical management of otitis media

Generic (Trade)	Frequency	Pediatric Daily Dosage	Comments
First-line antibiotic therapy			
Amoxicillin (Amoxil)	TID	40 mg/kg/day	Still the drug of choice for initial therapy
High dose amoxicillin	TID	80–90 mg/kg/day	Use first line if high incidence of penicillin-resistant pneumococcus
Trimethoprim-sulfamethoxazole, (Bactrim; Septra)	BID	1 tsp/10 lb body wt	When child is allergic to penicillin
Second-line antibiotic therapy			
Amoxicillin-clavulanate (Augmentin)	TID	40 mg/kg/d of amoxicillin	Broad spectrum, but 15% to 20% gastrointestinal upset
High-dose amoxicillin-clavulanate	BID	80–90 mg/kg/d of amoxicillin	Combine amoxicillin and amoxicillin clavulanate. Dose simultaneously. Keep clavulanate < 10 mg/kg/d
Azithromycin (Zithromax)	QD	10 mg/kg/day 1; 5 mg/kg/days 2–5	Suspension can be given without regard to food; capsules cannot
Cefprozil (Cefzil)	BID	30mg/kg/d	Not approved before 6 months of age
Cefpodoxime (Vantin)	QD	10 mg/kg/d	Broad spectrum, convenient dosing
Ceftibuten (Cedax)	QD	9 mg/kg/d	Broad spectrum, convenient dosing
Cefuroxime (Ceftin)	BID	30 mg/kg/d	Broad spectrum but bitter taste
Clarithromycin (Biaxin)	BID	15 mg/kg/d	Broad spectrum, well tolerated
Loracarbef (Lorabid)	BID	30 mg/kg/d	Must give 1 hour ac or 2 hours pc
Third-line antibiotic therapy			
Clindamycin (Cleocin)	TID	8–12 mg/kg/d	Superb for resistant pneumococcus
Ceftriaxone (Rocephin)	QD	50–75 mg/kg/d IM	Useful for refractory acute otitis media. May need to use 3-day course for resistant pneumococcus
Prophylactic antibiotics			
Amoxicillin (Amoxil)	QD	20 mg/kg/d	Must refrigerate; refill every 2 weeks
Sulfisoxazole (Gantrisin)	QD	30–75 mg/kg/d	No refrigeration necessary

Abbreviations: ac, before meals; pc, after meals; bid, twice daily; QD, once daily; TID, three times daily..

Adapted from Dowell SF et al. Acute otitis media: management and surveillance in an era of pneumococcal resistance—a report from the Drug-resistant *Streptococcus pneumoniae* Therapeutic Working Group. *Pediatr Infect Dis* 1999;18:1; and Rosenfeld RM. An evidence-based approach to treating otitis media. *Pediatr Clin North Am* 1996;43:1165.

fails, consider referral and possible tympanocentesis. If antibiotic resistance is prevalent, earlier tympanocentesis may be warranted.

Once the symptoms resolve, the child can ordinarily be rechecked after 4 to 6 weeks. Effusions are commonly seen during follow-up visits. In fact, 10% of children will have persistent effusions 3 months after acute otitis media. These children have **otitis media with effusion** (see later).

MANAGEMENT OF OTITIS MEDIA WITH EFFUSION

Parents of children with otitis media with effusion should be reassured (see AAFP Patient Ed Handout) and the children should be followed serially. If the effusion persists for 3 months, a hearing test is recommended, regardless of the child's age. If that test shows a reduction in hearing to 20 decibels in the better ear, a course of antibiotics like that for acute otitis media may be tried. Reduction of exposure to passive smoke, food, or other allergens or removal from day care may facilitate resolution. In addition, concurrent illnesses, such as allergic rhinitis or sinusitis, should be treated. If this is ineffective, referral for tympanostomy tubes is recommended. If the effusion persists without hearing loss, examination, including audiometry, every 3 or 4 months has been recommended (Rosenfeld).

MANAGEMENT OF RECURRENT ACUTE OTITIS MEDIA

Recurrent acute otitis media is defined as three or more distinct and well-documented episodes in the past 6 months or four episodes in the preceding year. If this definition is met, continuous antibiotic prophylaxis with amoxicillin, sulfamethoxasole or trimethoprim-sulfamethoxazole has been shown to decrease the rate of recurrence, although theoretically a child would need to be treated for 9 months to avoid one episode of acute otitis media (Rosenfeld). Children on antibiotic prophylaxis have an increased risk of bacterial resistance. Prophylaxis only during acute illnesses is less effective than continuous treatment. The risk of acute otitis media may be reduced by vaccinating against influenza A, eliminating passive smoke exposure, reducing day care attendance, and reducing pacifier use. If antibiotic prophylaxis is used, its use should be limited to no more than 6 months. Tympanostomy tubes are also effective in preventing recurrent otitis media. They should be strongly considered if a child has febrile seizures, hearing loss, speech problems, Down syndrome, craniofacial abnormalities, or immunodeficiency.

REFERRAL

Children who appear toxic—including those with poor eye contact, lethargy, very high fever, or signs of sepsis—should be seen by an otolaryngologist for possible typanocentesis. Consultation should also be obtained when mastoiditis or intracranial infection is suspected. Tympanostomy tubes may be needed for recurrent acute otitis

T ABLE 3.3.   Care of the child with tympanostomy tubes

Child may shower and bathe normally
Fitted ear plugs should be worn if the child dunks his head under bath water
Ear plugs are not needed for pool surface swimming
Fitted ear plugs should be worn for diving and underwater swimming, especially in lakes, ponds, or rivers

Adapted from text in Isaacson.

media or persistent otitis media with effusion. Table 3.3 outlines the care of the child with tympanostomy tubes. Of note, most episodes of otorrhea in children with tympanostomy tubes are related to upper respiratory tract infection and not to water exposure. Also, according to Salata, prophylactic ear drops or fitted ear plugs have not been shown to decrease the risk of otorrhea in children with tympanostomy tubes.

REFERENCES

Bredfeldt RC. An Introduction to tympanometry. *Am Fam Physician* 1991;44:2113.

Dowell SF, et al. Acute otitis media: management and surveillance in an era of pneumococcal resistance. A report from the Drug-Resistant *Streptococcus pneumoniae* Therapeutic Working Group. *Pediatr Infect Dis J* 1999;18:1.

Dowell SF, et al. Otitis media: principles of judicious use of antimicrobial agents. *Pediatrics* 1998;101:165.

Dowell SF, Phillips WR. Appropriate use of antibiotics for URIs in children. Part I: Otitis media and acute sinusitis. *Am Fam Physician* 1998;58:1113.

Isaacson G, Rosenfeld RM. Care of the child with tympanostomy tubes. *Pediatr Clin North Am* 1996;43:1183.

Kozyrskyj AL, et al. Treatment of acute otitis media with a shortened course of antibiotics: A meta-analysis. *JAMA* 1998;279:1736.

Maxson S, Yamauchi T. Acute otitis media. *Pediatr Rev* 1996;17:191.

Otitis Media Guideline Panel of the American Academy of Pediatrics. Managing otitis media with effusion in young children. *Pediatrics* 1994;94:766.

Rosenfeld RM. An evidence-based approach to treating otitis media. *Pediatr Clin North Am* 1996;43:1165.

Salata JA, Derkay CS. Water precautions in children with tympanostomy tubes. *Arch Otolaryngol Head Neck Surgery* 1996;122:276.

Weiss JC, Yates GR, Quinn LD. Acute otitis media: making an accurate diagnosis. *Am Fam Physician* 1996;53:1200.

Patient Education

Otitis media. Handout available from AAFP online at www.familydoctor.org.

Pharyngitis

CHIEF COMPLAINT

"My child has a sore throat."

HISTORY OF PRESENT ILLNESS

When evaluating the child with a sore throat, the family physician should assess the severity and duration of pain as well as the presence of associated symptoms such as fever, chills, cough, rhinorrhea, headaches, swollen glands, myalgias, and gastrointestinal upset. Contact with others infected with proved strep throat or mononucleosis should be ascertained. Foreign travel and consumption of wild game are predisposing factors for uncommon causes of pharyngitis.

MEDICAL HISTORY

A history of recurrent strep pharyngitis or immunosuppression may change the evaluation and management.

PHYSICAL EXAMINATION

Trismus, drooling, ashen color, and maintaining the "sniffing position" are signs of possible airway compromise. Patients with these symptoms may require emergent management. As examination may worsen airway compromise, the pharynx of these children should not be inspected. In more ordinary sore throat, the focused examination includes the temperature, weight, eyes for icterus or conjunctivitis, ears, neck for adenopathy, lungs, heart, abdomen for organomegaly, and skin for rashes. In the mouth, palatal petechiae, pharyngeal or tonsilar erythema and exudate, thrush, and ulcerations should be noted.

DIFFERENTIAL DIAGNOSIS

In the usual case of childhood pharyngitis the differential diagnosis includes viral pharyngitis versus Group A beta-hemolytic streptococcal infection (GABHS). Generally, the child with GABHS has a fever, rapid onset of symptoms, and a lack of rhinorrhea and cough. On examination the posterior pharynx is erythematous and may have a patchy exudate. There may be tender anterior cervical adenopathy and a sandpaper-like rash. Unfortunately, these findings are not specific for GABHS pharyngitis, and so the diagnosis should not be made on clinical grounds alone. On the other hand, GABHS is rarely the cause of pharyngitis associated with a low-grade or no fever, cough, rhinorrhea, conjunctivitis, and prolonged scratchy throat. Mononucleosis is caused by Epstein-Barr virus (EBV) or the cytomegalovirus. These children, often adolescents, present with fever, malaise, and pharyngitis, usually with exudate. Other less common causes of pharyngitis are listed in Table 3.4.

LABORATORY TESTING

In general, **GABHS** should not be diagnosed without laboratory confirmation. The rapid streptococcal antigen detection tests have a specificity when compared with throat culture of 90% to 96%; therefore clinically, a positive rapid strep indicates GABHS infection. There are false-negatives (sensitivity 76% to 87%), so a negative test requires confirmation with a culture if clinical suspicion exists. Both tonsilar pillars and the posterior pharynx should be swabbed. The throat culture is the gold standard for the diagnosis of GABHS. Use of a bacitracin disk diminishes false-positive results

T ABLE 3.4.   Less common causes of pharyngitis

Disease	Comments
Gonococcus	Adolescents, oral genital exposure
Diphtheria	Following foreign travel, especially to the former Soviet Union
Tularemia	Rabbit hunters, following a tick bite
Hand, foot, and mouth	Coxsackievirus, painful vesicles or ulcers on pharynx
Postnasal drip	Accompanying allergic rhinitis or sinusitis

with strep from groups other than Group A. Of note, the standard throat culture detects only GABHS, so the laboratory must be notified if other pathogens are suspected. A positive ASO titer confirms streptococcal infection in the previous months. This test is usually not useful in acute pharyngitis. If **mononucleosis** is suspected, atypical lymphocytes on CBC or a positive monospot may confirm infection. In the first week of infection or in children less than 4 years of age, the monospot is often false negative. In these cases EBV serology may be needed for diagnosis.

MANAGEMENT

Antibiotics have been shown to decrease the duration of symptoms and the risk of rheumatic fever following GABHS (Table 3.5). Penicillin remains the first-line therapy.

T ABLE 3.5. Antibiotics for confirmed GABHS pharyngitis (10-day course unless specified)

Medication	Frequency	Dosage	Comments
First line			
Benzathine penicillin	Once	25,000 U/kg, maximum 1.2 million U	Intramuscular, eliminates noncompliance
Penicillin V	Two or three times a day	25–50 mg/kg/d	First line, poor taste, narrow spectrum
Erythromycin estolate	Two times a day	20 mg/kg/d	For penicillin-allergic patients may cause jaundice
Erythromycin ethylsuccinate	Two times a day	40 mg/kg/d	For penicillin-allergic patients
Second line			
Amoxicillin (Amoxil)	Three times a day	40 mg/kg/d	Better tasting. Best for concurrent otitis media
Amoxicillin-clavulanate (Augmentin)	Two times a day	45/mg/kg/d of amoxicillin	High cost. Superior bacteriologic eradication
Azithromycin (Zithromax)	Once a day	12 mg/kg/d	5-day regimen. Different dose from otitis media. Fewer GI side effects than erythromycin
Cefuroxime axetil (Ceftin)	Two times a day	20mg/kg/d	Poor taste. 4–10-day course
Cefpodoxime proxetil (Vantin)	Two times a day	10 mg/kg/d	Poor taste. Chocolate syrup or strawberry yogurt "chaser" may help. 5–10-day course
Cefprozil (Cefzil)	Two times a day	15 mg/kg/d	Better tasting
Cephalexin (Keflex)		Two times a day	25–50 mg/kg/d
Clindamycin (Cleocin)	Three times a day	20–30 mg/kg/d	Risk of pseudomembranous colitis

Adapted from Pichichero ME. Group AB hemolytic streptococcial infections. *Pediatr Rev* 1998;19:291.

Erythromycin is the recommended alternative in penicillin-allergic patients. Other effective choices include the newer macrolides and cephalosporins. To decrease the incidence of antibiotic resistance, widespread use of broader-spectrum, second-line agents should be avoided. However, these agents may be particularly effective when compliance is difficult or in recurrent infection. The cephalosporins show more effective eradication of GABHS from the throat than penicillin. In most cases antibiotic treatment should be withheld until laboratory confirmation is available. If the clinician chooses to treat GABHS with antibiotics while the throat culture is pending, the supply of antibiotics should be limited to 2 days, with additional antibiotics prescribed once the culture is positive. Patients should be made aware that compliance with the full antibiotic course is crucial for the reduction in risk of rheumatic fever. Delay of initiation of antibiotic therapy has not been shown to increase the risk of rheumatic fever.

Antibiotics are not beneficial in viral pharyngitis. Treatment of viral pharyngitis is supportive and includes analgesics such as acetaminophen or ibuprofen and topical anesthetics. Treatment of mononucleosis is also supportive. Contact sports should be avoided until hepatosplenomegaly resolves. An abdominal ultrasound may be advisable before allowing return to very-high-contact sports such as football. Corticosteroids are recommended only in the setting of airway compromise or other severe complications such as massive splenomegaly.

REFERRAL

Tonsillectomy has traditionally been considered if the patient has six GABHS infections in 1 year or three or four infections in each of two successive years, although evidence of benefit from tonsillectomy from rigorous, randomized controlled trials is not available (Burton). Streptococcal toxic shock syndrome presents with profound hypotension, shock, and multiorgan failure. The WBC and platelet count are usually depressed, whereas serum creatinine and creatinine kinase are elevated.

REFERENCES

American Academy of Pediatrics. Group A streptococcal infections. In: Peter G, ed. *1997 Red Book: report of the Committee on Infectious Diseases*, 24th ed. Elk Grove Village, IL: American Academy of Pediatrics, 1997:483.

Burton MJ, et al. Tonsillectomy versus non-surgical treatment for chronic/recurrent acute tonsillitis (Cochrane Review). In: The Cochrane library, issue 3, 1999. Oxford Update Software.

Dowell SF, Schwartz B. Appropriate use of antibiotics for URI's in children: Part II. Cough, pharyngitis and the common cold. *Am Fam Physician* 1998;58:1335.

Perkins A. An approach to diagnosing the acute sore throat. *Am Fam Physician* 1997;55:131.

Peter J, Ray CG. Infectious mononucleosis. *Pediatr Rev* 1998;19:276.

Pichichero ME. Group A beta-hemolytic streptococcal infections. *Pediatr Rev* 1998;19:291.

Pichichero ME. Sore throat after sore throat: Are you asking the critical questions? *Postgrad Med* 1997;101:205.

Ruoff GE. Recurrent streptococcal pharyngitis. *Postgrad Med* 1996;99:211.

Patient Education

Sore throat. Handout available from AAFP online at www.familydoctor.org.

Conjunctivitis

Conjunctivitis is a common infection in children. It typically presents with a red eye, discharge from one or both eyes, and crusting of the eye overnight. Purulent discharge is more common in bacterial infection than viral, but lack of purulence does not rule out a bacterial infection. The most common pathogens in infectious conjunctivitis are *H. influenzae, S. pneumoniae* or adenovirus. Infection can be spread by direct contact, large droplets, or fomites. Contact lens wearers are prone to pseudomonas infection and corneal injury including abrasion and ulceration. Itchy eyes especially in conjunction with other signs and symptoms of allergic rhinitis imply an allergic etiology. With a history of trauma, corneal abrasion must be considered.

On examination, the conjunctiva are usually injected with palpebral and bulbar edema. Inspection beneath the upper lid is indicated if a foreign body is considered. Fluorescein staining can be used to assess for corneal abrasion or ulceration. Preauricular lymphadenopathy is common in viral infection. Vesicles are seen in herpetic infection. As bacterial conjunctivitis is commonly associated with otitis media, sometimes without ear symptoms, the ears should always be examined. The remainder of the examination excludes concurrent illness. Culture is only needed in very severe infection or in cases that are refractory to the usual treatment.

TREATMENT

Treatment of conjunctivitis has been shown to lead to quicker resolution of symptoms and to be associated with greater bacterial eradication (Lohr). Although not specifically assessed, this eradication should lead to decreased bacterial transmission. Topical antibiotics are effective (Table 3.6). Ointments may be easier to instill in a young uncooperative child than drops. Topical steroids should not be used without a slit lamp examination to rule out herpetic infection. Children may return to school when the discharge resolves and the eye is no longer discolored.

In the contact lens wearer, fluorescein staining may be needed to rule out an abrasion. As pseudomonas infection is common, antibiotics with gram-negative coverage (gentamicin [Garamycin, Genoptic]) and tobramycin [Tobrex]) are preferred. Contact lenses should not be worn until the infection clears completely, and they should be replaced or disinfected before use is resumed.

Allergic conjunctivitis usually responds to topical antihistamine/decongestant drops (Table 3.6).

Urgent ophthalmologic referral is indicated if herpetic infection is suspected, in a contact lens wearer with an abrasion or severe symptoms, or for very severe infection.

REFERENCES

Datner EM, Jolly BT. Pediatric ophthalmology. *Pediatr Clin North Am* 1995;13:669.

Giglotti F. Acute Conjunctivitis in childhood. *Pediatr Ann* 1993;22:353.

Lohr JA. Treatment of conjunctivitis in infants and children. *Pediatr Ann* 1993;22:359.

TABLE 3.6. Selected topical preparations for acute conjunctivitis

Medication	Treatment	Comments
For Bacterial Infection		
Polymyxin/Bacitracin (Polysporin)	Ointment: apply every 3–4 hours	
Sodium sulfacetamide,	Drops: 1–2 drops every 2–3 hours	
10% (Bleph-10, Sulamyd)	Ointment four times daily and at bedtime	
Polysporin/Bacitracin/Neomycin	Drops: 1–2 drops every 4 hours	
(Neosporin)	Ointment, every 3–4 hours	
Gentamicin (Garamycin, Genoptic)	Drops: 1–2 drops every 4 hours	Use more frequently for severe infection
	Ointment, two or three times daily	Use especially when gram-negative infection is suspected.
Tobramycin 0.3% (Tobrex)	Drops: 1–2 drops every 4 hours	Use more frequently for severe infection
	Ointment, two or three times daily	Use especially when gram-negative infection is suspected.
For Allergic Conjunctivitis		
Cromolyn sodium (Colom)	Drops: 1–2 drops every 4–6 hours	Not for use with soft contacts
Naphazoline (Vasocon)	Drops: 1–2 drops four times daily	
Naphazoline/Pheniramine (Naphcon A)	Drops: 1–2 drops four times daily	Nor for use with contact lenses

Sinusitis

Sinusitis is a common complication of upper respiratory infections, and with children experiencing three to eight viral upper respiratory infections annually, these infections are seen commonly by family physicians. Contrary to prior teaching, the maxillary and ethmoid sinuses are present at birth, although they are very small. The frontal and sphenoid sinuses appear at 5 or 6 years of age but may be only fully developed by adolescence.

Criteria have been developed to distinguish sinusitis from a viral upper respiratory infection (URI). These are

1. Signs of upper respiratory infection, including cough and nasal congestion, lasting more than 10 to 14 days without improvement.
2. More severe upper respiratory infection, which usually includes fever greater than 39°C, facial swelling, or facial or dental pain.

The first criterion is met most commonly when sinusitis is diagnosed. The amount or quality of nasal discharge, including thick, purulent discharge, does not distinguish a viral infection from a bacterial one. Chronic sinusitis is defined as the preceding symptoms lasting greater than 30 days. Abnormal sinus radiographs or CT scans may be seen in viral infections and are not diagnostic.

HISTORY

The history should include the duration and quality of the nasal discharge, and presence of fever (typically low grade). Facial and dental pain are rarely seen but imply more severe infection. Many children with sinusitis have malodorous breath. Cough is usually worse at night, but daytime cough is more indicative of sinusitis. Any history of recent antibiotic use or recurrent sinus infections should be elicited. Use of over-the-counter medications should be explored. Sinusitis is more common in children who attend day care or school.

PHYSICAL EXAMINATION

The temperature should be taken. Examine the eyes for swelling or decreased extraocular movement, which implies more severe disease. Transillumination is not helpful. Sinuses are rarely tender, except in early severe disease. If nasal polyps are present, cystic fibrosis should be ruled out. Otitis media frequently occurs with sinusitis. The remainder of the examination excludes concurrent illness.

LABORATORY EVALUATION

Laboratory testing is rarely needed. In the case of severe or persistent infection or in the immunocompromised host, aspiration of the sinus for gram stain and culture may be needed.

RADIOGRAPHY

Radiographic evaluation is rarely needed. If done early in the course of an uncomplicated upper respiratory infection, radiographs commonly show signs of bacterial sinusitis when it is not present. CT scans show more detailed information but are also rarely needed. No radiographic findings are specific for sinusitis in the absence of a clinical history indicative of sinusitis. Normal sinus films or CT scans, however, make bacterial sinusitis very unlikely. In children, especially those less than 1 year of age, an opacification of an undeveloped sinus may be misinterpreted as sinusitis.

TREATMENT

Once bacterial sinusitis is diagnosed by history and physical examination, antibiotic treatment is very effective. Amoxicillin (Amoxil) at 40 to 60 mg/kg/day is the first-line agent. Table 3.7 lists indications for use of other agents.

Drugs to treat sinusitis are listed in Table 3.8. When beta lactamase production is common, amoxicillin clavulanate (Augmentin) should be considered. When penicillin resistance is common, the dose of amoxicillin should be increased to 90 mg/kg/day. If the child does not respond within 48 hours of antibiotic use, the agent should be changed. Culture may be needed in severely ill children or those not responding to treatment. In general, antibiotics are continued for 10 days, although if the response was delayed, a 7-day course after the patient is asymptomatic may be prudent. Intranasal steroids may be helpful, especially with an underlying allergy. Antihistamines and oral or topical decongestants are not well studied and are unlikely to be helpful.

Hospitalization is reserved for those with very severe disease, such as orbital or central nervous system involvement, or those not able to take oral antibiotics.

CHRONIC AND RECURRENT SINUSITIS

Allergy, cystic fibrosis, immune deficiency, or structural abnormalities should be considered in a child with recurrent or chronic infection. If no underlying abnormality is found, prophylactic antibiotics, such as for otitis media, may be considered.

REFERRAL

Acute referral to an otolaryngologist is appropriate for very severe disease or if culture is needed. Later referral should be considered for resistant or recurrent disease. Enlargement of the ostial window has been shown to be effective, whereas nasoantral windows probably are not. Adenotonsillectomy may be beneficial if enlargement is causing obstructing clearance of secretions from the sinus.

T ABLE 3.7.   Indications for agents other than lower-dose amoxicillin

Amoxicillin allergy
Failure to improve on amoxicillin
Treatment with amoxicillin in the past month
High prevalence of beta lactamase—producing *H. influenzae* or *M. catarrhalis*
Frontal or sphenoid sinusitis
Complicated ethmoid sinusitis
Greater than 30 days of symptoms

Adapted from Wald ER. Sinusitis. *Pediatr Ann* 1998;27:811.

T ABLE 3.8. Recommended drugs for medical management of sinusitis

Antibiotic	Frequency	Pediatric Daily Dosage	Comments	Red Book Cost
First-line antibiotic therapy				
Amoxicillin (Amoxil)	3 times a day	40 mg/kg/d	Still the drug of choice for initial therapy	
High-dose amoxicillin	3 times a day	80–90 mg/kg/d	Use first-line if high incidence of penicillin-resistant pneumococcus	
Trimethoprim-sulfamethoxazole (Bactrim; Septr)	2 times a day	1 tsp/10 lb body weight	When child is penicillin allergic	
Second-line antibiotic therapy				
Amoxicillin-clavulanate (Augmentin)	3 times a day	40 mg/kg/d of amoxicillin	Broad-spectrum, but 15% to 20% gastrointestinal upset	
High-dose amoxicillin-clavulanate	2 times a day	80–90 mg/kg/d of amoxicillin	Combine amoxicillin and amoxicillin clavulanate. Dose simultaneously. Keep clavulanate <10 mg/kg/d	
Azithromycin (Zithromax)	4 times a day		Suspension can be given without regard to food; capsules cannot	
Cefprozil (Cefzil)	2 times a day	10 mg/kg day 1; 5 mg/kg days 2–5	Not approved before 6 months of age	
Cefpodoxime (Vantin)	4 times a day	30 mg/kg/d	Broad-spectrum, convenient dosing	
Cefibuten (Cedax)	4 times a day	10 mg/kg/d	Broad-spectrum, convenient dosing	
Cefuroxime (Ceftin)	2 times a day	9 mg/kg/d	Broad-spectrum, but bitter taste	
Clarithromycin (Biaxin)	2 times a day	30 mg/kg/d	Broad-spectrum, well tolerated	
Loracarbef (Lorabid)	2 times a day	15 mg/kg/d	Must give 1 hour before meals or 2 hours after meals	
		30 mg/kg/d		

continued

TABLE 3.8. Recommended drugs for medical management of sinusitis *(continued)*

Antibiotic	Frequency	Pediatric Daily Dosage	Comments	Red Book Cost
Third-line antibiotic therapy				
Clindamycin (Cleocin)	3 times a day		Superb for resistant pneumococcus	
Ceftriaxone (Rocephin)	4 times a day	8–12 mg/kg/d 50–75 mg/kg/d IM	Useful for refractory acute otitis media. May need to use 3-day course for resistant pneumococcus	
Prophylactic antibiotics				
Amoxicillin (Amoxil)	4 times a day	20 mg/kg/d	Must refrigerate; refill every 2 weeks	
Sulfisoxazole (Gantrisin)	4 times a day	50–75 mg/kg/d	No refrigeration necessary	

Adapted from Dowell SF, et al. Acute otitis media: management and surveillance in an era of pneumococcal resistance—a report from the Drug-resistant *Streptococcus pneumoniae* Therapeutic Working Group. *Pediatr Infect Dis* 1999;18:1; Rosenfeld RM. An evidence-based approach to treating otitis media. *Pediatr Clin North Am* 1996;43:1165.

REFERENCES

Blumer J. Clinical perspectives on sinusitis and otitis media. *Pediatr Infect Dis* 1998;17:S68.

Isaacson G. Sinusitis in childhood. *Pediatr Otolaryngol* 1996;43:1297.

O'Brien KL, et al. Acute sinusitis: principles of judicious use of antimicrobial agents. *Pediatrics* 1998;101:174.

Wald ER. Sinusitis. *Pediatr Ann* 1998;27:811.

CHAPTER 4

Gastrointestinal Ailments

Gastroenteritis/Oral Rehydration

CHIEF COMPLAINT

"My child is vomiting and having diarrhea."

HISTORY

For many parents a single, loose stool is diarrhea, so the frequency, quantity, and type of bowel movements must be assessed, as should the duration of diarrhea and associated symptoms of fever and abdominal pain. Frequency of vomiting and ability to retain solids and liquids must be assessed, as should frequency and quantity of urination. The use of home remedies such as broths with high sodium content or Jell-O water, Kool-Aid, sodas, and apple juice with low sodium is associated with electrolyte abnormalities. The presence of blood in either diarrhea or vomitus suggests more severe illness. Exposure to others with similar complaints makes an infectious etiology likely. A history of foreign travel or immunosuppression makes less common causes of gastroenteritis more likely.

Table 4.1 lists historical elements and associated causes of gastroenteritis.

PHYSICAL EXAMINATION

The physical examination begins with measurement of vital signs and weight. If a recent weight on the same scale is available, these weights can be used to determine the percent dehydration. The main goal of the physical examination is to assess the state of hydration. Table 4.2 lists methods for assessing degree of hydration. This scale may underestimate the dehydration if the child is hypernatremic. The abdominal examination should be used to rule out masses, organomegaly, or an acute abdomen. The presence of petechiae should be noted.

T ABLE 4.1. Historical elements and associated causes of gastroenteritis

History	Possible Association
Exposure to contaminated water from wells, streams, or lakes	Giardia
Exposure to turtles or undercooked poultry	Salmonella
Recent antibiotic use	Clostridium difficile
New infant formula	Formula intolerance

T ABLE 4.2.   Assessment of dehydration

Mild (5% to 6%)
Increased thirst, slightly dry mucous membranes, no other signs

Moderate (7% to 9%)
Signs of mild dehydration plus skin turgor change, sunken eyes or fontanelle, very dry mucous membranes

Severe (>9%)
Signs of moderate dehydration plus altered sensorium, rapid or weak pulse, cold extremities

From Goepp JG, Katz SA. Oral rehydration therapy. *Am Fam Physician* 1993;47:843.
Reprinted by permission.

LABORATORY ASSESSMENT

In the child with mild dehydration laboratory evaluation is generally unnecessary. Stool culture may be appropriate in a child with bloody diarrhea, high fever, or toxic appearance. The clinician needs to be aware of which pathogens are detected by the laboratory's standard stool culture and discuss specialized cultures if an unusual pathogen is suspected. Electrolytes, BUN, and creatinine are often necessary in the child who is more than 5% dehydrated or if home remedies with low or high sodium content have been used. The CBC is useful if the child appears toxic, for bloody diarrhea, or if petechiae are present.

DIFFERENTIAL DIAGNOSIS

Most acute gastroenteritis in children is viral in origin. In general, management does not depend on the exact infecting pathogen. The skin of children with hypernatremic dehydration tends to feel doughy instead of the usual tenting with isotonic dehydration. Ingestion of hypertonic solution during the illness is the usual inciting factor. Children with hypernatremic dehydration need to be rehydrated more cautiously, as they are at risk of neurologic damage, and so this differential is of particular importance.

MANAGEMENT

The child with gastroenteritis with **no dehydration** should continue an age-appropriate diet. Breastfeeding is especially helpful, as the milk often contains protective antibodies. Lactose-containing formulas may be continued. Extra fluids should be offered but not forced. Rehydration fluid is not needed, although it may be used to replace the losses from the vomiting or diarrhea. Home remedies such as coke syrup or high- or low-sodium-containing fluids listed earlier should be avoided. If desired, the child may be given 10 mL/kg of rehydration fluid for each diarrheal stool. Table 4.3 lists the electrolyte content of rehydration solutions and home remedies. If up to **5% dehydration** is present, oral rehydration should be instituted, unless there are signs of an acute abdomen or intestinal obstruction. Parents should give the child oral rehydration solution (Rehydralyte, Pedialyte) at a rate of at least 1 teaspoon (5 mL) per minute using a teaspoon, syringe, or calibrated bottle. Dehydration will be corrected by 50 mL/kg plus ongoing losses given over 2 to 4 hours. Ongoing losses are calculated as 10 mL/kg for each diarrheal stool and the estimated volume of any emesis. The child may be allowed to drink more than 1 teaspoon per minute but, to avoid gas-

T ABLE 4.3. Comparison of oral rehydration solutions

Solutions	Composition			
	Glucose (g/dL)	Sodium (mEq/L)	Potassium (mEq/L)	Chloride (mEq/L)
Commercial solutions				
WHO solution	2.0	90	20	80
Hydra-Lyte	1.2	84	10	59
Rehydralyte	2.5	75	20	65
Pedialyte	2.5	45	20	35
Generic pediatric solution*	2.5	45	20	35
Lytren	2.0	50	25	45
Resol	2.0	50	20	50
Infalyte	2.0	50	20	40
Ricelyte	Starch polymers	50	25	45
Home remedies (not recommended)				
Jell-O (one-half strength)	8.0	6 to 17	0.2	—
Gatorade	5.0	24	3	17
Soft drinks	7.0 to 12.0	1 to 7	0.1 to 0.4	—
Apple juice	12.0	0.1 to 3.5	24 to 43	—
Broth	—	250	—	—

Abbreviation: WHO, World Health Organization.

*Similar to Pedialyte.

From Eliason BC, Lewan RB. Gastroenteritis in children: principles of diagnosis and treatment. *Am Fam Physician* 1998;58:1769. Reprinted by permission.

tric distension, should not be allowed to "chug" large volumes of fluid quickly. In the dehydrated child, taste is less often an issue than when rehydration fluid is used in the nondehydrated child, but the fluid may be more palatable cold, flavored, or as a Popsicle. Vomiting does not preclude oral rehydration, as some fluid continues to be retained despite the vomiting, especially when small volumes are given frequently. As soon as the dehydration is corrected, the child should resume an age-appropriate diet. Many parents continue the rehydration fluid for prolonged periods if not specifically instructed not to do this.

Moderate dehydration may also be treated with oral rehydration. In this case the child is treated with 80 mL/kg of rehydration fluid with ongoing losses replaced as indicated earlier. Rehydration of these children generally is done in a supervised setting, such as the office, hospital, or emergency room, and a log is kept to record oral intake as well as ongoing losses. Criteria for failure of oral rehydration include increasingly negative fluid balance during rehydration, worsening signs of dehydration, or failure to rehydrate after 8 hours.

Antidiarrheal and antiemetic medications are usually not helpful. The use of empiric antibiotics is not recommended. If the child has severe diarrhea with fever, or blood or leukocytes in the stool, antibiotic treatment may be indicated, depending on the infecting organism.

REFERRAL

Referral is rarely needed for gastroenteritis. Children with greater than 10% dehydration are generally treated with intravenous fluids and hospitalization. Similarly, children who fail oral rehydration may need hospitalization. The evaluation of chronic diarrhea varies from this and may require the assistance of a gastroenterologist.

REFERENCES

Eliason BC, Lewan RB. Gastroenteritis in children: principles of diagnosis and treatment. *Am Fam Physician* 1998;58:1769.

Goepp JG, Katz SA. Oral Rehydration Therapy. *Am Fam Physician* 1993;47:843.

Provisional Committee on Quality Improvement, Subcommittee on Acute Gastroenteritis. American Academy of Pediatrics. Practice parameter: the management of acute gastroenteritis in young children. *Pediatrics* 1996;97:424.

Patient Education

Vomiting and diarrhea in children. Handout available from AAFP online at www.familydoctor.org.

Constipation and Encoporesis

CHIEF COMPLAINT

"My child is soiling his underwear." "My child has trouble moving his bowels."

HISTORY

The evaluation begins with determining the age at onset of constipation as well as any psychosocial stressors occurring at the time the problem began. Frequency and size of bowel movements, including toilet plugging; the presence of fecal or urinary incontinence; or urinary tract infections should be ascertained. Abdominal or anal pain or decreases in appetite should be noted. The child should be asked what he or she thinks causes the soiling and about any fears regarding using the toilet, especially in public places. Parents may mistake soiling for diarrhea and treat the child with antidiarrheal medications that worsen the constipation.

Past Medical History

A history of previous constipation or toilet-training difficulties should be explored. Chronic medical problems—including neurologic abnormalities of the gut, obstructive conditions of the colon, or endocrine problems—may lead to constipation.

Family History

Hirschsprung's disease, cystic fibrosis, hypothyroidism, neurofibromatosis, and myopathies may be familial and may cause constipation. Parental difficulties with constipation should be explored.

Social History

Fecal soiling can provoke great anger in parents. The response of the parents and child to the soiling should be assessed, as well as the effect on peer interactions. Family stressors should be discussed.

PHYSICAL EXAMINATION

Nutritional status and growth should be assessed. On abdominal examination, fecal masses may be felt in the left lower quadrant. The neurologic examination should emphasize perianal sensation and reflexes. The rectal examination assesses the presence of fissures or impacted stool and the size of the rectal vault. Some authors suggest deferring the rectal examination when the history is classic, to emphasize the child's own control of his or her own body and avoid discomfort. The remainder of the examination assesses the general health of the child to rule out other conditions presenting as constipation.

DIFFERENTIAL DIAGNOSIS

By far most children presenting to the family physician with constipation have functional constipation. These children will otherwise appear well, and the history will include stool withholding. Hirschsprung's disease occurs in one in 25,000 children, and the constipation usually begins in the newborn period. Hirschsprung patients rarely have fecal incontinence and usually pass small-caliber stools. They rarely have palpable stool in the vault. Many other metabolic and intestinal diseases may result in constipation. In general, these processes will be evident from the history and physical. Children who do not respond to routine management of constipation may need reevaluation and consideration of less common conditions.

LABORATORY TESTS

In general, laboratory and radiologic testing is not needed for the diagnosis of functional constipation. At times an abdominal flat plate may be shown to the child and parents to demonstrate the retained stool. If Hirschsprung's disease or another uncommon cause of constipation is suspected, specialized evaluations may be needed.

MANAGEMENT

The management of functional constipation begins with an explanation of the problem to both child and parents. Specifically, they need to understand that the buildup of stool leads to distension of the colon. Once this occurs, future bowel movements are large and painful, and liquid stool may leak out. Parents need to empathize with the child's embarrassment and work with the child toward resolution. The diet should include adequate quantities of fluid and fiber. Helpful foods include fruits and vegetables, prune juice, and bran cereal. Constipating foods, such as milk, apples, and bananas, should be avoided. A bowel routine may be established by having the child sit on the toilet for 10 minutes once each day, generally after a meal. A foot stool may facilitate the Valsalva maneuver. Reading may make this time more pleasant for the child. Whenever the child feels the urge to defecate, he or she should be allowed to use the toilet, especially in school. Positive reinforcement can be especially helpful. Children should keep a calendar and record a star for successful bowel movements. These charts can be brought to office visits.

Pharmacologic intervention may be needed if the preceding measures fail or at the onset if the problem has been longstanding. Bulk-forming agents are usually tried first. If these are ineffective, emollient agents or lactulose may be tried. Resistant cases may require stimulants (Table 4.4).

T ABLE 4.4. Suggested dosages of laxatives commonly used to treat constipation in children

Agent	Child's Age	Dosage
Bulk-forming laxatives		
Psyllium	6 to 12 years	2.5 g one to four times daily
	>12 years	5 g one to four times daily
Malt soup extract	Breast-fed infants	5–10 mL in 2 to 4 oz of water two times daily
	Bottle-fed infants	5–10 mL in every second feeding
Emollient laxatives		
Mineral oil	>6 months	2 mL/kg daily in one to two divided doses
Docusate sodium	<3 years	10–40 mg daily in two to three divided doses
	3 to 6 years	20–60 mg daily in two to three divided doses
	7 to 12 years	40–120 mg daily in two to three divided doses
	>12 years	50–200 mg daily in two to three divided doses
Saline laxatives		
Magnesium sulfate or magnesium hydroxide	>6 months	2 mL/kg daily in one to two divided doses
Sodium phosphate/ biphosphate enema	2 to 12 years	Children's enema, 2.5 oz
	>12 years	Adult's enema, 4.5 oz
Stimulant laxatives		
Senna syrup	1–5 years	2.5–5 mL at bedtime
	6–15 years	5–10 mL at bedtime
Bisacodyl tablets or suppository	6–12 years	5 mg at bedtime
	>12 years	10 mg at bedtime
Hyperosmotic laxatives		
Lactulose	>6 months	Concentration of 10 g per 15 mL: 1–2 mL per kg daily in two to three divided doses
Glycerine suppository	<1 year	0.7 g suppository
	1–6 years	1–1.5 g suppository

From Leung AK, Chan PY, Cho HY. Constipation in Children. American Family Physician. 1996;54:611. Reprinted by permission.

T ABLE 4.5. Disimpaction regimen

Day 1	Two hypophosphate enemas
Day 2	Dulcolax suppository twice daily
Repeat for two to four cycles until the impaction resolves	

From Zuckerman B. Encoporesis. In: Parker S, Zuckerman B, eds. *Behavioral and developmental pediatrics.* Boston: Little, Brown, 1995:125.

T ABLE 4.6. Disimpaction enemas

Mineral oil	2 ounces per 10 kg up to 4.5 oz
Hypertonic phosphate	1 ounce per 10 kg up to 4.5 oz
Milk and molasses	50:50 mix up to 6 ounce maximum

From Abi-Hanna A, Lake AM. Constipation and encoporesis in childhood. *Pediatr Rev* 1998;19:23.

If the stool is impacted, enemas may be required (Tables 4.5 and 4.6). If this regimen is not effective, mineral oil or milk and molasses enemas may be tried. If the stool remains impacted, pulsed rectal irrigation or oral lavage may be needed (Abi-Hanna). Once the stool is disimpacted, regular toileting, as discussed earlier, and stool softeners are employed.

REFERRAL

Referral is rarely needed for functional constipation. If other entities are suspected, the need for referral depends on the individual physician's level of expertise. At times, functional constipation may be the result of severe psychopathology and psychiatric referral may be needed.

FOLLOW-UP

Early in the management process, weekly follow-up visits are often needed. As the child improves, the interval between visits is extended. If medications were needed in the treatment, they should be weaned gradually. Parents should be advised to have the child seen at the first signs of recurrence. Once the acute problem is resolved, the frequency and difficulty of bowel movements can be assessed during well-child and other visits.

REFERENCES

Abi-Hanna A, Lake AM. Constipation and encopresis in childhood. *Pediatr Rev* 1998; 19:23.

Leung AK, Chan PY, Cho HY. Constipation in children. *Am Fam Physician* 1996;54: 611.

Rudolph C, Benaroch L. Hirschsprung disease. *Pediatr Rev* 1995;16:5.

Zuckerman B. Encoporesis. In: Parker S, Zuckerman B, eds. *Behavioral and developmental pediatrics.* Boston: Little, Brown, 1995:125.

Patient Education

Constipation in children. Handout available from AAFP online at www.familydoctor.org.

CHAPTER 5

....

Orthopedic Concerns

Special Considerations of the Pediatric Knee

Orlando F. Mills

The child's knee has growth plates on the distal femur and proximal tibia. Both growth plates are evident at birth and completely ossify by 20 years of age. The growth plates are considerably weaker than the surrounding ligaments. When the knee is damaged by trauma, the growth plate is more likely to be injured than the collateral or cruciate ligaments. As the child gains skeletal maturity and participates in high-impact sports, the risk of ligament damage increases. The physician examining a child or adolescent with a painful knee should consider injury to the growth plate. Fractures through the growth plate are described by the Salter-Harris classification, as shown in Fig. 5.1.

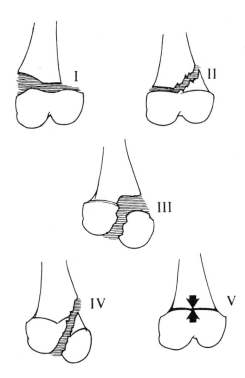

FIGURE 5.1. The Salter-Harris classification of fractures involving the growth plate. (From Sponseller PD. Bone, joint, and muscle problems. In: McMillan JA, DeAngelis CD, Feigin RD, Warshaw JB, eds. *Oski's pediatrics: principles and practice.* New York: Lippincott Williams & Wilkins, 1999.)

HISTORY

The initial symptoms of a knee problem are pain, stiffness or swelling in the adolescent or preadolescent child, and a limp in the younger child. The infant, toddler, and early-school-age child rarely present with knee pain unless there is a traumatic, infectious, or neoplastic origin. In the case of trauma, the mechanism of injury helps direct the examination. If the event is not consistently described, child abuse may be suspected. The child with an infectious origin for a knee problem may or may not have evidence of minor trauma to the knee, followed by a limp or refusal to walk and evidence of systemic illness. The child with a neoplastic knee lesion may present with limp or refusal to walk and localized pain and swelling. The adolescent or preadolescent may also have an infectious or neoplastic process that affects the knee, but this is uncommon. The family physician should recognize that knee pain in the school-aged child may be caused by hip pathology. Finally, a normal knee examination in the setting of continued knee pain or a limp may represent a functional knee disorder in which the limb pain indicates psychosocial distress in the child.

PHYSICAL EXAMINATION

The examining physician searches for problems in the function of the knee, its supporting structures, and attachments. The complete knee evaluation includes a measurement of leg lengths because markedly disparate leg lengths can cause a dysfunctional gait with a limp or knee pain. If possible, the child's gait should be observed for pain during the stance phase (antalgic gait). The physician inspects, palpates, and tests range of motion of the knee with the child in the supine position. The physician observes the knee for swelling, erythema, or loss of normal landmarks. Swelling seen above or lateral to the patella may represent an effusion, whereas swelling below the patella may represent prepatellar bursitis, and swelling behind the knee may be a popliteal cyst. The physician judges a knee effusion by placing one hand on the knee superior to the patella (compressing the suprapatellar pouch) and pressing to the side of the knee, observing for the movement of fluid. In a confirmatory but less sensitive test, the physician presses the patella gently downward, and if the patella is depressible there may be a joint effusion. Loss of the normal concavity to the side of the knee may also indicate a joint effusion.

The physician examines both knees when testing the integrity of the ligaments and cartilage. The normal knee is used as a reference during the examination. The physician palpates the joint line formed by the tibial plateau and the distal femur. Tenderness at the medial or lateral joint line may indicate a medial or lateral meniscal tear, or injury to the lateral collateral ligaments. The physician tests the integrity of the collateral ligaments by holding the knee with one hand and placing a varus or valgus stress on the ankle/foot (Fig. 5.2). During varus stress, in which pressure is exerted from the lateral side of the ankle, the lateral collateral ligament will be stretched. The lower leg adducts slightly in the normal leg but will be felt to adduct excessively in the partially or completely torn lateral collateral ligament. In addition, the completely torn lateral collateral ligament will not have a "firm endpoint"; the knee does not resist further adduction until this is limited by pain or apprehension. Valgus stress on the knee abducts the lower leg and tests the integrity of the medical collateral ligament and the medial meniscus, which are anatomically connected.

The physician tests the anterior cruciate ligament (ACL) and posterior cruciate ligament (PCL). The Lachman test is performed with the knee in 10° to 15° of flexion. The physician places one hand on the upper tibia with the thumb on the joint line and places the other hand on the middle to lower thigh. After asking the child to relax the muscles of the leg, the physician holds the thigh still and pulls the lower leg ante-

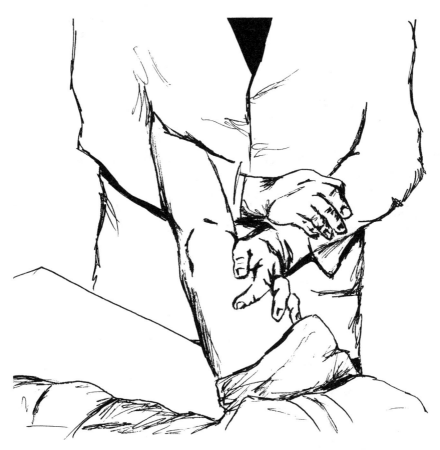

FIGURE 5.2. Valgus stressing of the MCL is applied by stabilizing the limb between the elbow and the trunk. The left hand is placed on the lateral aspect of the distal femur and the right hand is stabilized by grasping the left forearm.

riorly. Anterior motion of the lower leg greater than 1 or 2 cm may indicates a partially or completely torn ACL. The ACL may also be tested with the leg flexed 90°. The physician sits gently on the child's foot, pulls the lower leg anteriorly, and looks for excessive forward motion (anterior drawer test) (Fig. 5.3). The posterior drawer test involves pushing the tibia posteriorly with the knee bent 90°. Excessive posterior displacement of the tibia indicates PCL laxity or a partial or complete tear.

The patella is examined for tenderness and stability. The physician gently displaces the patella medially, then laterally, and palpates the undersurface of the patella for tenderness. The patella is displaced inferiorly and the child is asked to tighten the thigh (leg extension). Inability to do so reflects inflammation of the patellar undersurface (positive patellar inhibition sign). The examiner attempts to displace the patella laterally, and if this is resisted it indicates a subluxing patella (positive patellar apprehension sign).

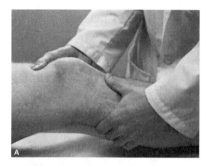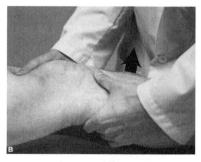

FIGURE 5.3. The Lachman test. With the patient supine, the knee is flexed to 20° to 30°. **A:** While the femur is stabilized with one hand, the tibia is grasped with the other hand. **B:** When pulled anteriorly in the absence of the anterior cruciate ligament, the tibia moves excessively anteriorly. (From Landry GL. Sports medicine. In: McMillan JA, DeAngelis CD, Feigin RD, Warshaw JB, eds. *Oski's pediatrics: principles and practice.* New York: Lippincott Williams & Wilkins, 1999.)

IMAGING STUDIES

The most important imaging study of the injured knee is the plain radiograph, which should include at least three views: anteroposterior, lateral, patellar, and/or tunnel view (with 30°, 60°, or 90° of flexion). The plain radiograph demonstrates the presence of normal alignment of bony structures and growth plates and can exclude a fracture of the patella, distal femoral condyles or proximal tibial plateau. The magnetic resonance imaging (MRI) study of the knee may have very good sensitivity (80% to 100%) and specificity (89% to 95%) for meniscal tears in children, but it is rarely needed in the evaluation of most pediatric knee injuries.

LABORATORY TESTING

Laboratory testing, including culture and cell count of the synovial fluid, is needed, especially if a septic joint is suspected.

DIAGNOSIS AND MANAGEMENT

Table 5.1 lists the diagnosis and management of common pediatric knee problems.

REFERENCES

Al-Otaibi L, Siegel MJ. The pediatric knee. *Magn Reson Imaging Clin N Am* 1998;6: 643.

Behrman RE, ed. *Textbook of pediatrics.* Philadelphia: WB Saunders, 1992:1703.

Davids JR. Pediatric knee: clinical assessment and common disorders. *Pediatr Clin North Am* 1996;43:1067.

Ramamurti CP. Orthopedics in primary care. Baltimore: Williams & Wilkins, 1984:187.

Roach JW. Knee disorders and injuries in adolescents. *Adolesc Med* 1998;9:589.

Stanitski CL. Pediatric and adolescent sports injuries. *Clin Sports Med* 1997;16:613.

TABLE 5.1.   Common pediatric knee conditions

Condition	History and Physical Examination	X-ray/Imaging	Treatment/Comments
Meniscal tear	Meniscal tear in young child suggests lateral discoid meniscus. Adolescent in competitive sports may injure knee when foot is planted and leg rotates suddenly or is hit from side. May feel pop in knee with possible effusion, joint line tenderness near meniscal tear. If cartilage is loose, knee may lock.	Plain films useful to exclude fracture. Three views with tunnel view (if condyles tender) or skyline view (if possible patellar fracture). MRI generally unnecessary.	Consider orthopedics referral. Conservative therapy with NSAIDs, rest, strengthening. Arthroscopy for locked knee or persistent pain.
Discoid meniscus	Most common congenital abnormality of meniscus. Affects lateral meniscus, which is thicker medially than normal meniscus. Can tear with knee flexion. Possible pain/limp with clunk at joint line when knee is flexed.	Plain films to exclude other disorders. MRI images meniscus and shows abnormality.	Conservative treatment. Arthroscopy for persistent pain or effusion.
ACL tear	May occur in adolescents, with female predominance. In complete ACL tear, athlete feels a "pop." Effusion evolves immediately or in a few hours. Knee feels unstable—walking difficulty initially. May occur with medial meniscal tear.	Plain films generally done to exclude osteochondral fracture, if clinician in doubt.	Initially, weight bearing with knee brace, then quadriceps strengthening with resumption of reduced sporting activity with knee brace if added stability needed. Rehabilitative process takes weeks to months. Surgery postponed until full skeletal maturity is reached.
Medial collateral ligament tear	Uncommon before physis closes. Child instead would have injury to tibial/femoral physis. Child with skeletal maturity may have partial/complete tear of collateral ligament. Pain and knee instability seen on affected side. Examine for integrity of sciatic nerve and popliteal artery.	Films used to rule out fracture of epiphysis, femoral or tibial condyles.	Refer promptly if sciatic nerve or popliteal artery injury. Rest and gradual weight bearing, leg strengthening if not complete tear. Full tear suspected: Examine for ACL tear and refer to orthopedics if present.

Abbreviations: ACL, anterior cruciate ligament tear; MRI, magnetic resonance imaging; NSAIDs, nonsteroidal antiinflammatory drugs.

Problems of the Pediatric Hip

Orlando F. Mills

PRESENTING HISTORY

The physician suspects a pediatric hip problem when the child refuses to walk or bear weight on the affected leg, complains of pain in the knee or hip, or walks with a limp. Because both the hip and knee are innervated by the obturator nerve, hip problems may present as knee pain. The physician asks about the onset and duration of symptoms and inquires about congenital hip anomalies, recent trauma, fever, viral infections or diarrhea, steroid use, or sickle cell disease.

PHYSICAL EXAMINATION

The physician examines the child while she lays on her back on a firm table. The physician assesses hip flexion by bringing the thigh to the chest. The hip and knee are bent to 90°, and the physician tests internal rotation by rotating the lower leg outward and tests external rotation by rotating the lower leg inward (Fig. 5.4). The examiner tests abduction with the hip flexed with the leg straight. Both knees and hips are flexed 90°, and the leg is rotated outward, testing abduction. Next, both legs are straightened, and each leg is abducted again. The physician observes the child's gait. In the antalgic (painful) gait, the child decreases the time spent bearing weight on the affected side because of pain. The child with a Trendelenburg gait bears weight on the affected side but then leans to the opposite side and swings the affected leg forward because of abductor muscle weakness.

LABORATORY EVALUATION

In most cases, an x-ray of the hip is needed for evaluation. Comparison views of the unaffected leg may be useful. If septic hip is considered a complete blood count, sedimentation rate or culture of the hip aspirate may be needed.

DIFFERENTIAL DIAGNOSIS

The differential diagnosis of hip problems includes infections (septic arthritis, Lyme disease, osteomyelitis, iliopsoas abscess), inflammatory conditions (juvenile rheumatoid arthritis, Lyme disease, rheumatic fever), tumors (neuroblastoma, Ewing's sarcoma, osteogenic sarcoma, osteoid osteoma), trauma, and overuse syndromes. In the following sections some of the more common and important hip ailments in children are discussed.

Congenital Dislocation of the Hip
See Chapter 2.

Septic Arthritis
The child with a septic hip is generally 3 years of age or younger and develops fever (80% of the time), refuses to walk, or walks with a limp and appears acutely ill. The hip is maintained in a flexed, frog-leg position and cannot be moved easily on exam-

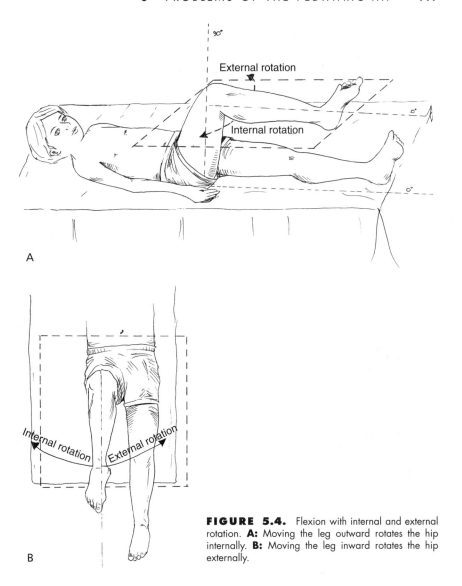

External rotation

Internal rotation

A

Internal rotation   External rotation

B

FIGURE 5.4. Flexion with internal and external rotation. **A:** Moving the leg outward rotates the hip internally. **B:** Moving the leg inward rotates the hip externally.

ination. The white blood cell count (WBC) and erythrocyte sedimentation rate (ESR) are elevated, and the x-ray may show soft-tissue swelling. The physician who suspects a septic hip should obtain an orthopedics consultation for urgent hip aspiration. The common bacterial pathogens in a septic hip are staphylococcus, pneumococcus, group A streptococcus, *Neisseria meningitidis,* group B streptococcus (if <6 months), salmonella species (sickle cell patient), or *Haemophilus influenzae* (if not immunized). Appropriate antibiotic therapy should be instituted after hip aspiration. Delayed treatment of the septic hip can lead to avascular necrosis or arthritis.

Transient (or "Toxic") Synovitis

Typically, the patient with transient synovitis is 3 to 5 years of age, has a 1- to 2-week onset of discomfort in the knee or hip, limps, and may have a low-grade fever. Though viral pathogens are presumed, transient synovitis has no known etiology. On examination, the child maintains the hip in flexion, resists rapid movement of the hip, and limits the range of motion. The WBC, ESR, and hip x-ray are usually normal. The child with transient synovitis may be initially hospitalized and placed on bedrest. As the child improves, non–weight-bearing ambulation with crutches is advised. When the child has painless, full motion of the hip, he or she may resume full weight bearing. The differential diagnosis of transient synovitis includes septic arthritis and avascular necrosis of the hip (Perthes' disease). Septic arthritis can usually be excluded by the lack of fever, toxicity, and elevated WBC count, but if there is any doubt, the child is referred to orthopedics for hip aspiration. Transient synovitis is differentiated from Perthes' disease by hip x-rays, which may need to be repeated if hip pain does not resolve.

Perthes' Disease

In Perthes' disease the blood supply to the femoral head is interrupted, leading to necrosis of the femoral head. The reason for this circulatory disruption generally is not known. The age range is 3 to 10 years, with a peak incidence between 5 and 10 years of age. The avascular section of the femoral head is eventually reabsorbed by granulation tissue. Subsequently, the femoral head is remodeled over a period of 2 to 2.5 years. The child with Perthes' disease has a gradual onset of pain in the groin, knee, or hip that becomes more prominent with activity and is reduced by rest. The child has an intermittent limp because of the pain. On examination, the child keeps the hip in some degree of flexion, may have a flexion contracture, and has pain with abduction, internal rotation, and extension of the hip. An x-ray performed 2 months or more after the onset of symptoms will show increased density of the involved hip; x-rays months later will show mottling and distortion of the femoral head. Bone scanning shows decreased uptake of the femoral head, and MRI demonstrates avascular necrosis. If Perthes' disease is strongly suspected, the family physician should refer the patient to orthopedics for bracing, casting, or osteotomy. The objective of these treatments is to keep the femoral head well centered in the acetabulum during the phase of bone remodeling. The prognosis for the child with this disease is best when the child presents at a young age and with intact range of motion; the prognosis is the least favorable in the older child who presents with a restricted range of motion.

Slipped Capital Femoral Epiphysis

The child with a slipped capital femoral epiphysis (SCFE) sustains a slippage of the capital femoral epiphysis posteriorly and inferiorly. The typical patient is an obese male 10 to 14 years of age with thigh or knee pain of several weeks duration and an antalgic gait. SCFE also occurs in children who are unusually tall and slender and in girls (40% of cases). Most cases of SCFE are idiopathic, but a few are associated with hypothyroidism, growth hormone administration, renal osteodystrophy, or radiation therapy. SCFE affects both hips in 25% to 40% of the cases and may be *stable* or *unstable*. The stable slippage occurs gradually, in contrast to the unstable slippage, which occurs acutely after sports or other trauma. As the physician examines the child with a stable SCFE and attempts to flex the child's hip, the child externally rotates and abducts the hip to avoid painful internal rotation. The child may also walk with the affected foot pointed outward. The child with an unstable SCFE may refuse to allow any movement of the hip because of extreme pain. The diagnosis is made by anteroposterior (AP) and frog leg views of the hip. In the unstable SCFE, the only possible x-ray may be a single AP view of the hip. The physician who suspects or diagnoses a case of SCFE should refer the child to orthopedics for evaluation and surgical stabilization of the femoral head. If the diagnosis is in doubt, the physician should advise non-weight bearing pending complete evaluation. Avascular necrosis occurs in one-third or fewer cases of unstable slippage and less often in the stable slippage. Chondrolysis, degeneration of the articular cartilage, may complicate the clinical course in 5% to 7% of all cases.

REFERENCES

Hart JJ. Transient synovitis of the hip in children. *Am Fam Physician* 1996;54:1587.

Loder RT. Slipped capital femoral epiphysis. *Am Fam Physician* 1998;57:2135.

Ramamurti CP. Orthopedics in primary care. Baltimore: Williams & Wilkins, 1984:187.

Richards BS. Slipped capital femoral epiphysis. *Pediatr Rev* 1996;17:69.

Shaw BA, Gerardi JA, Hennrikus WL. How to avoid orthopedic pitfalls in children. *Patient Care* Feb 1999; 33(4)95.

Theophilopoulos EP, Barrett DJ. Get a grip on the pediatric hip. *Contemp Pediatr* 1998;15:43.

Patient Education

Slipped capital femoral epiphysis. Handout available from AAFP online at www.familydoctor.org.

CHAPTER 6

Urologic Concerns

Bed-wetting

CHIEF COMPLAINT

"My child wets the bed."

HISTORY OF PRESENT ILLNESS

The evaluation of a child with enuresis should include the onset of bed-wetting, the frequency, and the number of episodes per month. Any history of daytime or fecal incontinence should be elicited. A voiding history should include frequency of daytime voiding, daytime dribbling, difficulty in starting or stopping stream, and longest period of daytime continence.

PAST MEDICAL HISTORY

Any past history of central nervous system trauma, urinary tract infection, other urologic abnormalities, diabetes, sleep apnea, or seizure disorder would direct the workup. Children with behavioral problems are more likely to be bed-wetters.

FAMILY HISTORY

In families where both parents were enuretic, 70% of children wet the bed, whereas when only one parent was affected, 40% of children have enuresis. A family history of urologic disorders should be obtained.

SOCIAL HISTORY

Psychosocial stressors are an important etiology, especially for secondary enuresis (enuresis after being dry for 6 months). Stressors such as parental divorce, school problems, or abuse occurring at the time the child began wetting are especially important. Procedures for cleaning the bed and child following the incidents should be explored. Unfortunately, some families punish and embarrass bed-wetters, which may worsen the problem.

PHYSICAL EXAMINATION

During the physical examination particular attention should be paid to the neurologic examination, specifically to gait abnormalities, and strength and deep tendon reflexes in the lower extremities. The sacral area should be inspected for dimpling or skin changes suggestive of spinal pathology. If the history indicates, the urinary stream should be observed and a rectal examination performed. A distended bladder or genital abnormalities should be noted. In general, however, the physical examination will be unrevealing.

LABORATORY EVALUATION

For most children a urinalysis and culture are the only laboratory evaluations needed. Other tests, including imaging studies, are done only when suggested by the history or physical.

DIFFERENTIAL DIAGNOSIS

More than 97% of children evaluated for bed-wetting have physiologic enuresis. Boys have a greater incidence than girls. At 5 years of age, 20% of children wet the bed monthly. This declines to 10% by age 6 and to 15% per year thereafter. Other causes may be suggested by the history and physical examinations and include detrusor muscle instability, polyuria, and incomplete bladder emptying or filling.

TREATMENT

Treatment depends on the age of the child. Parents of 3- or 4-year-olds need to be reassured and advised that this is physiologic and not misbehavior. Beyond this age, behavioral interventions should be started (Table 6.1).

If these simple interventions are ineffective and the child is at least 6 years old, a positive reinforcement system can be set up. A monthly calendar placed on the refrigerator can be very effective. When the child stays dry, a sticker is placed on the corresponding day of the calendar. If the child awakened at night to use the toilet, a more special sticker can be used. Once the child earns five stickers, a reward can be given. The use of this system may be the parents' first introduction to positive reinforcement as a motivator. Before going to bed the child should be reminded to wake up and use the toilet when his bladder is full. Many children are unable to "hold it" all night. If the bed-wetting persists, the parents may awaken and toilet the child during the night.

Enuresis alarms either emit a harsh sound or vibrate when the child urinates. These alarms have a higher success rate than any other treatment for enuresis. The child should be told to wake himself up before the alarm sounds. Parents and patients must be motivated, and it may take 2 to 3 months for resolution. If the child does not awaken to the alarm, the parents should awaken him and bring him to the toilet.

If the preceding treatments are ineffective, medications may be tried. Table 6.2 lists the commonly used ones. Often the medications are most effective when combined with the behavioral techniques. After a few months of successful use, an attempt is made to taper the medication gradually. Unfortunately, the rate of relapse is significant.

T ABLE 6.1.   Behavioral interventions for the bed-wetting child

1. Avoid excessive fluid intake and caffeine 2 hours before bedtime
2. Improve nighttime access to the toilet (night light, portable toilet)
3. Empty the bladder at bedtime
4. Involve the child in the cleanup in a nonpunitive way
5. Preserve self-esteem by giving positive reinforcement, including for areas unrelated to bed-wetting.

Adapted from Schmitt BD. Nocturnal enuresis. *Pediatr Rev* 1997;18:183.

T ABLE 6.2.   Medications for enuresis

Medication	Initial Dose	Cost	Taper	Precaution/Comments
Desmopressin (DDAVP)	One spray (10 μg) each nostril at bedtime (maximum 40 μg/d)		One spray every 2 weeks	Hyponatremia possible with excessive fluid intake. Keep refrigerated
Imipramine (Tofranil)	8–12 years: 25–50 mg at bedtime >12 years: 50–75 mg at bedtime		25 mg every 2 weeks	Lethal in overdose. Keep away from small children
Oxybutynin (Ditropan)	6–12 years: 5 mg at bedtime >12 years: 10 mg at bedtime			Especially beneficial for small bladder capacity and urge incontinence

Used with permission from Schmitt BD. Nocturnal enuresis. *Pediatr Rev* 1997;18:183.

REFERRAL

Referral is suggested for the child with underlying neurologic abnormalities. Psychologic referral may be needed for families with severe stress or dysfunction. Referral may also benefit the older child who continues to have enuresis despite adequate trials of medication.

REFERENCES

Byrd RS, Weitzman M, Lanphear NE, Auinger P. Bed-wetting in US children: epidemiology and related behavior problems. *Pediatrics* 1996;98:414.

Schmitt BD. Nocturnal enuresis. *Pediatr Rev* 1997;18:183.

Ullom-Minnich MR. Diagnosis and management of nocturnal enuresis. *Am Fam Physician* 1996;54:2259.

Patient Education

Bed-wetting. Handout available from AAFP online at www.familydoctor.org.

Enuresis Alarms

Potty Pager. 800-497-6573. $51.95.

Nite Train-r. 800-544-4240. $69.

Hematuria

CHIEF COMPLAINT

"I was told my child has blood in his urine."

HISTORY

Despite recommendations against routine screening for hematuria, many children present following detection of blood in their urine. These urine tests may have been done routinely or may have been done as part of an evaluation of another condition such as fever. Usually the child is asymptomatic. Children also present, often franti-

T ABLE 6.3. Clues in the history and possible diagnosis

Characteristic	Possible Associated Condition
Brown or tea-colored urine	Glomerular lesion
Gross hematuria with viral illnesses	IgA nephropathy
7–21 days following strep pharyngitis or impetigo	Poststreptococcal glomerulonephritis
Dysuria, flank pain	Urinary tract infection, nephrolithiasis
Petechial/purpuric rash of lower extremities	Henoch-Schönlein purpura
Malar rash	Systemic lupus erythematosus
Edema	Glomerulonephritis
Hypertension	Glomerulonephritis
Vigorous exercise	Transient hematuria
Trauma, abuse	Transient hematuria

Used with permission from Fitzwater DS, Wyatt RJ. Hematuria. *Pediatr Rev* 1994;15:102.

cally, following an episode of gross hematuria. Then timing, frequency, and duration of the hematuria should be ascertained. Table 6.3 lists historic elements and their associated conditions.

PAST MEDICAL HISTORY

Children with sickle cell disease or trait, polycystic kidney disease, or systemic lupus erythematosus are prone to hematuria. Congenital heart disease may lead to endocarditis and hematuria associated with immune complex glomerulonephritis. Diuretics may cause hypercalcuria and subsequent hematuria. Especially following umbilical catheterization, newborns may develop hematuria from renal artery or vein thrombosis.

FAMILY HISTORY

A family history of deafness and renal failure, especially in males, suggests Alport's syndrome. Thin basement membrane disease, IgA nephropathy, and nephrolithiasis also have familial predispositions.

PHYSICAL EXAMINATION

Hypertension is a worrisome finding and should prompt an expedited evaluation. Edema may be most obvious in the periorbital area. Malformed ears are associated with congenital renal disease. Rales or gallops suggest fluid overload. Murmurs may suggest congenital heart disease. Abdominal masses may suggest polycystic kidneys, and renal bruits may be heard. Nephrosis may cause ascites. Costovertebral angle tenderness is seen in pyelonephritis and nephrolithiasis. The genitalia should be inspected for trauma. The skin should be examined for rashes, and extremities should be checked for edema and arthritis.

LABORATORY EVALUATION

Figure 6.1 outlines the laboratory evaluation of a child who presents with hematuria. If the history, including family history, or physical examination suggests a particular etiology, the laboratory evaluation should be individualized.

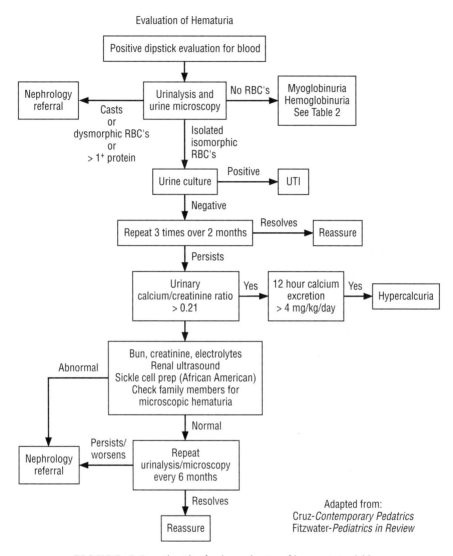

FIGURE 6.1. Algorithm for the evaluation of hematuria in children.

DIFFERENTIAL DIAGNOSIS

Multiple conditions can cause hematuria in the child. Poststreptococcal glomerulonephritis begins 7 to 21 days after group A beta-hemolytic strep infection. Children usually present with tea-colored urine, edema, and hypertension. The C3 is usually
depressed and the ASO is initially elevated. The microscopic hematuria usually resolves
by 12 months, with normal renal function after recovery. IgA nephropathy usually presents with gross hematuria associated with viral illnesses, usually without hypertension
and edema. Serum IgA levels may be elevated, but diagnosis can only be made by renal

biopsy. The prognosis varies from remission to chronic renal insufficiency. Alport hereditary nephrosis may present with gross hematuria associated with viral illness or even semicontinuous gross hematuria. Usually a family member with nerve deafness or end-stage renal disease can be identified. The syndrome is X-linked dominant. Renal biopsy confirms the diagnosis and assesses prognosis. Family members should be screened for hematuria and hearing impairment. Hypercalcuria may present with gross hematuria even in the absence of stones. The diagnosis is made by a spot urinary calcium/creatinine ratio greater than 0.21. This should be confirmed by a timed urinary calcium excretion of greater than 4 mg/kg/day. Following confirmation, a renal ultrasound should be done to rule out nephrolithiasis. Treatment involves increasing fluid intake and restricting salt intake. Calcium restriction has not been shown to be beneficial. Patients who are actively forming stones should be referred to a nephrologist for further management.

REFERRAL

Referral may be guided by the algorithm in Fig. 6.1. Early referral is recommended in very young children and in children with findings on history, physical examination, or urinalysis.

REFERENCES

Cruz CC, Spitzer A. When you find protein or blood in the urine. *Contemp Pediatr* 1998;15:89.

Fitzwater DS, Wyatt RJ. Hematuria. *Pediatr Rev* 1994;15:102.

Neiberger RE. The ABC's of evaluating children with hematuria. *Am Fam Physician* 1994;49:623.

U.S. Public Health Service. *Put prevention into practice: clinician's handbook of preventive services*, 2nd ed. McLean, VA: International Medical Publishing, 1998.

Proteinuria

CHIEF COMPLAINT

"I was told my child has protein in his urine."

HISTORY

Despite recommendations against routine screening for proteinuria, many asymptomatic children are found to have protein in their urine. These urinalyses may have been done routinely or as part of an evaluation of another condition such as fever. Usually the child is asymptomatic. Any history of recent streptococcal infection, hematuria, edema, change in urinary habits, dysuria, or unexpected change in weight should be elicited. It is important to be aware of previous renal disease, hypertension, or a family history of renal disease, including dialysis and transplant.

PHYSICAL EXAMINATION

The physical examination should include height, weight, and blood pressure. Signs of pallor, ascites, or edema should be noted. In young children the kidneys may be palpable.

LABORATORY EVALUATION

Figure 6.2 outlines the laboratory evaluation of a child found to have proteinuria. The first step in the evaluation is a repeat complete urinalysis, ideally on the first morning specimen. If two such specimens are free of protein, the patient should be reassured and further evaluation is unnecessary. Urine culture should be obtained if infection is suspected. If the proteinuria persists, orthostatic proteinuria should be ruled out by measurement of recumbent urinary protein excretion (Fig. 6.2). To do this, the child

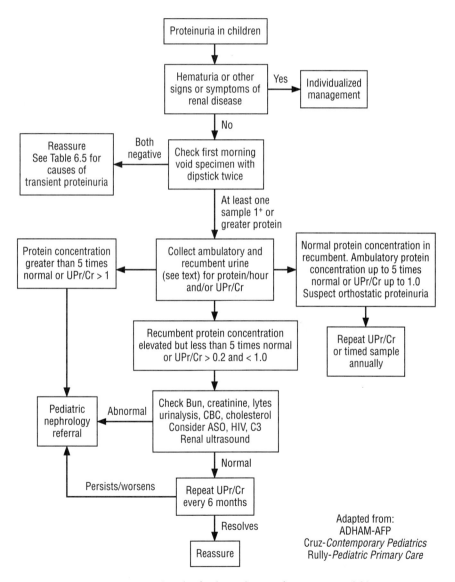

FIGURE 6.2. Algorithm for the evaluation of proteinuria in children.

T ABLE 6.4. Normal urinary protein excretion in children

Age	Total Protein (mg/d)	UPr/Cr
2–12 months	38	<0.5
2–4 years	49	<0.2
4–10 years	85	<0.2
10–16 years	63	<0.2

UPr/Cr, urinary protein to creatine ratio.
Used with permission from Miltenyi M. Urinary protein excretion in healthy children. *Clin Nephrol* 1979;12:216.

should void before going to bed, record the time, and discard the sample. Immediately upon awakening, the child should void, record the time, and save the specimen as "recumbent." The urine throughout the day should be collected and labeled "ambulatory." The final specimen before going to bed should be saved and the time should be recorded. As this process is difficult for patients and some samples may be lost, it may be preferable to collect the ambulatory specimen for part of the day and know the exact duration of the collection. One way to circumvent the difficulties with collecting a timed sample is the urinary protein-to-creatine ratio (UPr/Cr). This ratio is measured on random urine samples and correlates with the total protein excretion. Table 6.4 lists normal ranges for protein and UPr/Cr for various ages.

If the total protein remains elevated, other laboratory evaluation should include electrolytes, BUN, creatinine, albumin, and complete blood count. When poststreptococcal glomerulonephritis is suspected, an ASO titer should be added. Depending on the clinical presentation, evaluation for HIV or systemic lupus erythematosus may be indicated.

DIFFERENTIAL DIAGNOSIS

Tables 6.5 and 6.6 list the causes of false-positive urine dipstick results and transient proteinuria.

If the proteinuria persists, the most common cause is orthostatic proteinuria. In this condition, children, usually adolescents, spill protein while active but do not have proteinuria while recumbent. The prognosis is excellent. Other causes of proteinuria are much less common and are often diagnosed by a nephrologist following specialized testing.

T ABLE 6.5. Causes of transient proteinuria

Strenuous exercise
Exposure to extreme cold
Febrile illness
Seizure
Epinephrine exposure
Emotional stress
Congestive heart failure
Abdominal surgery

Used with permission from Cruz CC, Spitzer A. When you find protein or blood in the urine. *Contemp Pediatr* 1998;15:89.

T ABLE 6.6. Causes of false-positive urine dipstick results

White cells in the urine
Bacteriuria
Prolonged immersion of the strip
Extremely alkaline pH (pH > 8)
Heavy mucus
Semen
Detergents

Used with permission from Cruz CC, Spitzer A. When you find protein or blood in the urine. *Contemp Pediatr* 1998;15:89.

REFERRAL

Cellular casts or persistent hematuria warrant early referral to a nephrologist. Similarly, very young children or children with other signs or symptoms of renal disease should be referred early. Otherwise, referral can be guided by Fig. 6.2.

REFERENCES

Abitbol C, Zillerueldo G, Freundlich M, Strauss J. Quantitation of proteinuria with urinary/creatinine ratios and random testing with dipsticks in nephrotic children. *J Pediatr* 1990;116:243.

Cruz CC, Spitzer A. When you find protein or blood in the urine. *Contemp Pediatr* 1998;15:89.

Loghman-Adham M. Evaluating proteinuria in children. *Am Fam Physician* 1998;58:1145.

Ruley EJ. Proteinuria. In: Hoekelman RA. *Pediatric primary care,* 3rd ed. St Louis, MO: Mosby, 1997:1078.

U.S. Public Health Service. *Put prevention into practice: clinician's handbook of preventive services,* 2nd ed. McLean, VA: International Medical Publishing, 1998.

Patient Education

Proteinuria in children. Handout available from AAFP online at www.familydoctor.org.

Urinary Tract Infection

CHIEF COMPLAINT

"It hurts when my child urinates." "My child has a fever."

HISTORY OF PRESENT ILLNESS

Children vary in their presentation with urinary tract infection (UTI). Older children may complain of dysuria, frequency, urgency, or suprapubic pain, whereas younger children may have urinary incontinence or fever. Children with pyelonephritis may have flank pain, but not all do. An abnormal odor may be present. Constipation is associated with an increased risk of urinary tract infections, whereas breast feeding is associated with a diminished risk.

PAST MEDICAL HISTORY

Children with a previous urinary tract infection are prone to repeat infections. Abnormalities of the central nervous system also increase the risk. Children with preexisting voiding dysfunction as evidenced by urgency, frequency, dribbling, or incontinence are at increased risk. Uncircumcised infant males are at increased risk. Children with urinary calculi or vesicoureteral reflux are also at increased risk. Children with past or current hypertension may have this on the basis of renal scarring and should receive a radiologic evaluation after the first urinary tract infection, with early specialist referral.

FAMILY HISTORY

Children with a first urinary tract infection and a family history of urinary tract abnormalities should receive a radiologic evaluation.

PHYSICAL EXAMINATION

The physical examination should include measurement of temperature and blood pressure. Particular attention should be paid to abdominal masses, flank masses, or costovertebral angle tenderness, a palpable bladder, abnormal genitalia, pilonidal sinuses, or neurologic abnormalities.

LABORATORY EVALUATION

In children, urinary tract infection can only be reliably diagnosed with a positive urine culture, with the exception of the adolescent female with classic symptoms and a positive urinalysis. In young children this culture should be obtained with a catheterized specimen or suprapubic aspiration (especially in uncircumcised boys). Table 6.7 describes the technique for bladder catheterization.

In older toilet-trained children a midstream clean catch may be possible. Table 6.8 lists the criteria for a positive urine culture with the various collection techniques.

T ABLE 6.7.   Bladder catheterization

1. For children under 1 year of age use a no. 4 feeding tube; in children 1–6 years of age use a no. 6 feeding tube
2. For boys: Using sterile technique, straighten the urethra with gentle caudal traction and cleanse the urethral opening with 3 povidine-iodine swabs.
   For girls: Using sterile technique, separate the labia and expose the urethral opening. Cleanse from the clitoris toward the rectum using one swab for each labia and one for the center.
3. Slowly insert the catheter coated with a thin film of sterile lubricant into the urethra. Resistance will be noted at the external sphincter of the bladder. This will be overcome with continued pressure. (In girls the catheter will only need to advance a few centimeters.) Catch the first few drops in a separate sterile container and the rest in a second one.
4. Send the second container for culture (unless the first sample is all that is obtained).

Used with permission from Hoberman A, Wald ER. UTI in young children: new light on old questions. *Contemp Pediatr* 1997;14:140.

T ABLE 6.8.   Criteria for a positive urine culture

Collection Method	Positive Result
Suprapubic aspiration	Any colonies present
In-and-out catheterization	10^3 colonies
Midstream clean catch	10^5 colonies

Adapted with permission from Ahmed SM, Swedlund SK. Evaluation and treatment of urinary tract infections in children. *Am Fam Physician* 1998;57:1573.

Lower colony counts may be indicative of infection if repeated specimens yield the same organism or in the symptomatic child. Bagged urine specimens with fewer than 10^5 colonies in a child off antibiotics rule out a urinary tract infection. However, it is impossible to differentiate contamination from urinary tract infection in a bagged specimen or a specimen obtained from a diaper. In a sick child where antibiotics are being started immediately and therefore a follow-up urine culture before antibiotics will be impossible, a bagged specimen has little utility.

TREATMENT

Treatment of the child with a urinary tract infection depends on the age of the child and the severity of illness. Children less than 3 months of age and others who appear toxic or appear to have pyelonephritis are usually hospitalized and treated with parenteral antibiotics. Other children may be treated with oral antibiotics, usually for 10 days. Shorter courses of therapy are effective in adults and so are reasonable in adolescents, but they are not well studied in children. Table 6.9 lists the antibiotics commonly used for urinary tract infection in children.

FOLLOW-UP

The follow-up of a child following a UTI remains controversial. In fact, a recent review found that there are no controlled studies on diagnostic imaging following a urinary tact infection, and, furthermore, according to Dick, none of the studies provided evidence on clinical outcomes. In children, some urinary tract infections are complicated by renal parenchymal scarring. This scarring may lead to an increased risk of hypertension and renal failure. Unfortunately, this scarring may already be present

T ABLE 6.9.   Some oral antibiotics used in the treatment of urinary tract infection in children

Amoxicillin (Amoxil)	20–40 mg/kg/day divided in three doses
Cephalexin (Keflex)	50–100 mg/kg/day divided in four doses
Sulfisoxazole (Gantrisin)	120–150 mg/kg/day divided in four doses
Trimethoprim-sulfamethoxazole* (Bactrim, Septra)	6–12 mg TMP, 30–60 mg smx per kg per day in two doses

*Use cautiously in the first month of life because of risk of jaundice.

Used with permission from American Academy of Pediatrics. The diagnosis, treatment, and evaluation of the initial urinary tract infection in febrile infants and young children. *Pediatrics* 1999;103:843.

after the first urinary tract infection. Management strategies seek to minimize both the risk of long-term sequelae and that of invasive and expensive testing. Figure 6.3 outlines a management strategy for a child with a urinary tract infection. Of note, renal ultrasound has not been shown to detect all clinically significant reflux. Intravenous urography has little role in the workup of urinary tract infections in children, as it requires a higher dose of radiation and has a lower sensitivity for pyelonephritis and renal scarring than renal scintigraphy. Finally, surgical treatment of high-grade vesicoureteral reflux has been shown to offer no advantage when compared with medical management (antibiotic prophylaxis, regular voiding, avoidance of constipa-

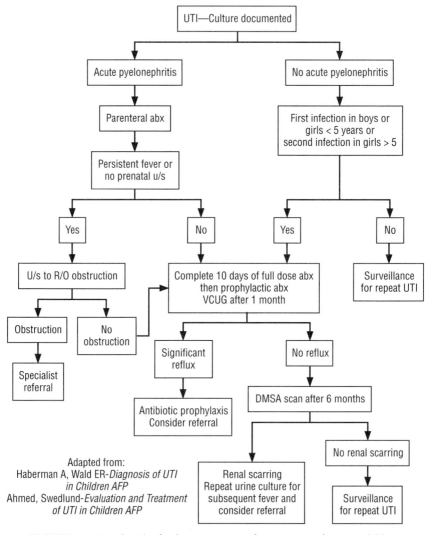

FIGURE 6.3. Algorithm for the management of urinary tract infection in children.

T ABLE 6.10. Antibiotics used for urinary tract infection prophylaxis

Nitrofurantoin* (Furadantin, Macrodantin)	1–2 mg/kg daily
Sulfisoxazole (Gantrisin)	10–20 mg/kg daily
Trimethoprim-sulfamethoxazole† (Bactrim, Septra)	2–4 mg TMP, 10 mg smx per kg as single bedtime dose, or 5 mg TMP, 25mg smx per kg twice per week

*Avoid in newborns or patients with renal insufficiency.
†Use cautiously in the first month of life because of risk of jaundice.
Used with permission from American Academy of Pediatrics: The diagnosis, treatment, and evaluation of the initial urinary tract infection in febrile infants and young children. *Pediatrics* 1999;103:843.

tion). Table 6.10 lists antibiotics commonly used for urinary tract infection prophylaxis.

REFERRAL

Urologic referral should be considered for significant reflux (grades III to V), renal scarring, or recurrent urinary tract infections (Fig. 6.3).

PATIENT EDUCATION

It has long been recommended that children with a history of urinary tract infection avoid bubble baths and at times even swimming. These interventions are of unproven benefit and should be avoided. Although wiping from front to back seems prudent, this too has not been of proven benefit. Constipation has been shown to increase the risk of urinary tract infection and should be managed aggressively. (See the section on constipation in Chapter 4.)

REFERENCES

Ahmed SM, Swedlund SK. Evaluation and treatment of urinary tract infections in children. *Am Fam Physician* 1998;57:1573.

Committee on Quality Improvement. Subcommittee on Urinary Tract Infection. American Academy of Pediatrics. Practice parameter: the diagnosis, treatment, and evaluation of the initial urinary tract infection in febrile infants and young children. *Pediatrics* 1999;103:843.

Dick PT, Feldman W. Routine diagnostic imaging for childhood urinary tract infections: a systematic review. *J Pediatr* 1996;128:15.

Eisenberg M. Critically Appraised Topic. Surgery vs medical management for high grade vesicoureteral reflux: pediatric evidence based medicine. December 1997. www.weber.u.washington.edu/ebm/

Hellerstein S. Urinary tract infections in children: why they occur and how to prevent them. *Am Fam Physician* 1998;57:2440.

Hoberman A, Wald ER. Diagnosis of urinary tract infection in children, editorial. *Am Fam Physician* 1998;57:2337.

Hoberman A, Wald ER. UTI in young children: new light on old questions. *Contemp Pediatr* 1997;14:140.

Ortigas AP, Cunningham AS. Three facts to know before you order a VCUG. *Contemp Pediatr* 1997;14:69.

Rushton HG. Urinary tract infections in children. Epidemiology, evaluation and management. *Pediatr Clin North Am* 1997;44:1133.

C HAPTER 7

Miscellaneous Concerns

Heart Murmur

CHIEF COMPLAINT

"I have been told my child has a heart murmur."

HISTORY OF THE PRESENT ILLNESS

Although the history rarely gives diagnostic clues to the exact cause of a heart murmur, it often helps determine the need for referral and the urgency with which that referral is needed. Specifically, any history of cyanosis—excluding normal peripheral cyanosis in a newborn, syncope, shortness of breath, exercise or feeding intolerance, or failure to thrive—is particularly important.

PAST MEDICAL HISTORY

Heart murmurs are more likely to be due to structural heart disease when the child has other congenital abnormalities or a history of prematurity. Also, heart disease is more likely if the pregnancy was complicated by the use of prescription medications, diabetes mellitus, illicit drugs, alcohol, or viral infections such as cytomegalovirus, herpes, or coxsackievirus.

FAMILY HISTORY

Because congenital heart disease runs in families, it is important to ask about heart disease, including hypertrophic cardiomyopathy or sudden cardiac death in siblings, parents, or other relatives.

PHYSICAL EXAMINATION

The growth chart is an essential part of the evaluation of a child with a heart murmur. Children with clinically significant heart disease often do not keep up with expected growth. For a child who is new to the practice this may require review of old records. On general examination the family physician should look for dysmorphic features and cyanosis. The blood pressure should be recorded with a cuff that covers two-thirds of the distance between the shoulder and antecubital fossa or the hip and popliteal fossa. In general, a cuff that is too large is better than one that is too small, because measurement with one that is too small can lead to overestimation of the systolic blood pressure. To rule out coarctation, the pressure is measured in both arms and one leg. In a young child this is best done using the flush method. To use the flush method, the uninflated blood pressure cuff is placed on the elevated arm. The fluid is then milked from the arm and the cuff is inflated above the estimated systolic pressure. The cuff is then deflated. The pressure where the arm flushes to match the other arm's color is midway between the systolic and diastolic pressure. Table 5 in the appendix gives the classification of hypertension based on age.

Auscultation of the back may reveal rales and murmurs, which are heard best posteriorly. Enlargement of the liver may be the only physical sign of congestive heart failure in children. On extremity examination, clubbing is a worrisome finding that may indicate heart disease. Pulses should be palpated, and if extremity pulses are diminished, the blood pressure should be recorded in all extremities.

Auscultation of the heart should be done at the time during the examination when the child is most cooperative, often at the beginning. Young children may be most cooperative clothed and on the parent's lap. The clinician should listen at the right upper sternal border, the left upper sternal border, the left lower sternal border, and the apex. The second heart sound should be split in children. This splitting widens with inspiration and diminishes with expiration. A fixed, or unchanging, split to the second heart sound is abnormal. If murmurs are heard, they should be characterized by the type of sound, intensity, loudest location, and radiation. Murmur intensity is graded on a scale of 1 to 6:

1. very soft
2. slightly louder
3. louder
4. loud with a palpable thrill
5. heard with stethoscope just off the chest
6. heard without stethoscope.

Table 7.1 lists the common innocent murmurs of childhood. Table 7.2 lists the common pathologic murmurs in childhood. Figure 7.1 depicts the location of the common murmurs.

WORKUP

The workup of a child with a heart murmur is determined by the findings on the history and physical examination. For a newborn with a murmur and signs of congestive heart failure, immediate consultation with a pediatric cardiologist is warranted. In a healthy child with a Still's murmur (see Table 7.1) on examination, no further workup is necessary. The chest x-ray can detect cardiomegaly and congestive heart failure. The electrocardiogram (EKG) can detect axis deviation, rhythm disturbances, and cardiac hypertrophy. Each of these tests should be used to confirm abnormalities detected on examination, and normal results do not exclude cardiac disease. Performance of echocardiography on a child requires pediatric expertise in both the technician and the interpreter. According to Hurwitz, echocardiograms performed on children by adult laboratories may be less adequate than those done in pediatric centers, and Danford points out that it is usually more cost-effective to refer patients to a pediatric cardiologist before ordering an echocardiogram. Echocardiography to "prove" that a murmur is innocent should be avoided. In cases of concerning murmurs, where pediatric cardiology services may be difficult to access or after consultation with a pediatric cardiologist, an echocardiogram may need to be ordered by a family physician. In these cases the family physician should verify that the test is being done properly and is interpreted by a cardiologist experienced in pediatric echocardiography for interpretation.

REFERRAL

Children with symptoms that do not meet the criteria for an innocent murmur should be evaluated by a pediatric cardiologist. In general, newborns should be evaluated

T ABLE 7.1. Innocent murmurs

Type	Typical Age	Symptoms	Sound	Location	Maneuver
Stills	Age 2–6	None	Vibratory Musical Intensity usually Grades 2 (1–3)	Left lower sternal border	Decreased intensity and changes pitch when upright
Pulmonary flow murmur	Children, adolescents, young adults	None	Crescendo—decrescendo Rough, dissonant Grades 2–3	Left upper sternal border (2nd & 3rd intercostal space)	Loudest supine with full exhalation (decreased intensity sitting, inhaling) distinguished from ASD-ASD has widely split S2 Pulmonary valve stenosis has ejection click
Venous hum	Age 3–8	Patient may hear loud "hum"	Humming, whining quality	Loudest low anterior neck, right greater than left	Louder sitting than lying Diminished by lying, turning head away from examiner
Supraclavicular Systolic murmur (Supraclavicular arterial bruit)	Children, young adults	None	Early systole	Above clavicles Radiates to neck more than chest	Eliminated by shoulder hyperextension

Based on data from: Allen HD, Golinko RJ, Williams RG. Heart murmur in children: When is a workup needed? *Patient Care.* 1994;123–151; Beerman LB, Fricker FJ, Park SC, Lenox CC. Cardiology. In: Zitelli BJ, Davis HW, eds. *Atlas of Pediatric Physical Diagnosis,* 3rd ed. Mosby-Wolfe, 1997:111–131; Pelech AN. The cardiac murmur. *Pediatr Clin North Am* 1998;45:107–122.

ASD, atrial septal defect.

TABLE 7.2. Common noninnocent murmurs

Type	Symptoms	Age	Sound	Location	Maneuver	Other
Ventricular septal defect	Usually asymptomatic; CHF when large	Infancy: Large defects. Later: Small to medium	Harsh systolic	Left lower sternal border	No change in sound with position. May have thrill	Many small defects close spontaneously in first year, may not need referral. Require SBE prophylaxis
Atrial septal defect	Usually asymptomatic; when large, CHF, decreased exercise tolerance	Childhood	Medium-pitched wide split	Left midsternal border. Left upper sternal border	RVI: palpable left sternal border	
Patent ductus arteriosus	Asymptomatic small; when large, CHF, poor growth	Ejection murmur Grades 1–3	Left infraclavicular; sometimes posterior radiation	Bounding pulses. May have thrill second left interspace		
Coarctation of aorta	Infants: Cardiovascular collapse. Older: Asymptomatic		Systolic murmur	Interscapular area. May be heard in third right intercostal space	Leg pulses weak and delayed compared with arms	Cause of hypertension in children
Hypertrophic cardiomyopathy (idiopathic hypertrophic subaortic stenosis)	None. Sudden cardiac death	Any age	Grades 2–3 systolic murmur. Often has no murmur	Murmur loudest at apex	Murmur intensified by standing after squatting. Increased by Valsalva	May have positive family history. Restrict from strenuous physical activity

Based on data from: Allen HD, Golinko RJ, Williams RG. Heart murmur in children: When is a workup needed? Patient Care 1994;123; Beerman LB, Fricker FJ, Park SC, Lenox CC. Cardiology. In: Zitelli BJ, Davis HW, eds. Atlas of pediatric physical diagnosis, 3rd ed. Mosby-Wolfe, 1997;111; Pelech AN. The cardiac murmur. Pediatr Clin North Am 1998;45:107.

CHF, congestive heart failure; SBE, subacute bacterial endocarditis.

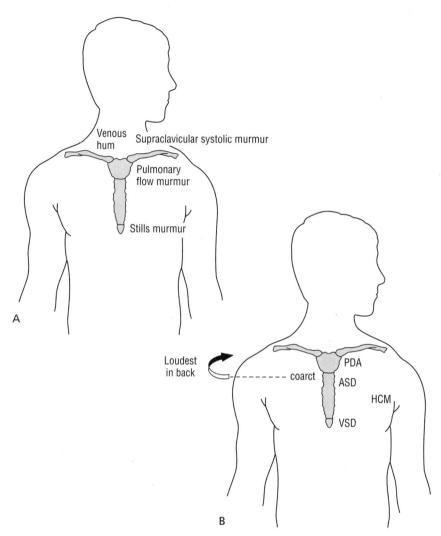

FIGURE 7.1. **A:** Location of common innocent murmurs. **B:** Location of common noninnocent murmurs. ASD, atrial septal defect; HCM, hypertrophic cardiomyopathy; PDA, patent ductus arteriosis; VSD, ventricular septal defect.

within hours, infants within days, and otherwise healthy children within weeks. A normal chest x-ray and EKG do not eliminate the need for referral, if the murmur does not fit the criteria for one of the innocent murmurs.

PATIENT EDUCATION

Children with innocent heart murmurs are at risk for the "vulnerable child syndrome." In this syndrome parents become overprotective of the child because of excessive concerns about the child's health. This may lead to the child developing behavioral problems. Family physicians need to reassure the parents that a child with an innocent murmur is "normal" and can participate in all normal activities, especially athletics. This should be reemphasized at subsequent visits. These children do not need antibiotic prophylaxis for subacute bacterial endocarditis.

Patient education for children with structural heart disease is generally reviewed by the pediatric cardiologist, although the family physician should verify that the parents have a good understanding of their child's condition.

REFERENCES

Allen HD, Golinko RJ, Williams RG. Heart murmur in children: when is a workup needed? *Patient Care* 1994;123.

American Academy of Pediatrics, Section on Cardiology. Echocardiography in infants and children. *Pediatrics* 1997;99:921.

Beerman LB, Fricker FJ, Park SC, Lenox CC. Cardiology. In: Zitelli BJ, Davis HW, eds. *Atlas of pediatric physical diagnosis,* 3rd ed. St Louis, MO: Mosby-Wolfe, 1997:111.

Danford DA, Nasir A, Gumbiner C. Cost assessment of the evaluation of heart murmurs in children. *Pediatrics* 1993;91:365.

Gutgesell HP, Barst RJ, Humes RA, Franklin WH, Shaddy RE. Common cardiovascular problems in the young: Part I. Murmurs, chest pain, syncope and irregular rhythms. *Am Fam Physician* 1997;56:1825.

Hurwitz RA, Caldwell RL. Should pediatric echocardiography be performed in adult laboratories? *Pediatrics* 1998;102:e15.

Leslie LK, Boyce WT. The vulnerable child. *Pediatr Rev* 1996;17:323.

Pelech AN. The cardiac murmur. *Pediatr Clin North Am* 1998;45:107.

Patient Education Resources

American Heart Association. Innocent murmurs. Heart and stroke A-Z guide. www.amhrt.org.

Seizures

Seizures have been defined as involuntary discharges of cortical neurons that may result in an impaired level of consciousness or in abnormal movement, sensation, or autonomic function. Febrile seizures are seizures in young children who have fever but no intracranial infection or history of nonfebrile seizures. Epilepsy refers to recurrent nonfebrile seizures.

HISTORY

In evaluating a child with a suspected seizure, the family physician must take a detailed history. What occurred during the event? For how long? Did it recur? Was the seizure focal or generalized? Did the child have any premonitory symptoms? Was the child incontinent of bowel or bladder? Was the child postictal? What was the child doing at the time of the event? Is there a history of trauma or ingestions? Is the child receiving any medication or using elicit drugs? Did the child have a fever before or after the event? If the child was febrile, the necessary history to evaluate the fever should be obtained. If the child has recurrent spells, the parents may be able to videotape the event.

PAST MEDICAL HISTORY

Has the child had similar events before? Is the child developing normally? Did the child have any neonatal complications? Does the child have other medical conditions?

FAMILY HISTORY

A family history of seizures, both febrile and afebrile, should be elicited. Is there a family history of unexplained syncope, including syncope with exercise or emotional upset, sudden infant death syndrome (SIDS), or drownings?

PHYSICAL EXAMINATION

Because a seizure may be secondary to an intracranial infection, the physician should consider this possibility and begin appropriate emergency evaluation and management if the child appears toxic or has meningeal irritation or other indicators of serious infection.

For evaluation of the seizure itself the physical examination should include the following:

Vital signs, including temperature

Complete neurologic examination

Developmental assessment
    If an absence seizure is suspected, a seizure may be brought on by voluntary hyperventilation for a few minutes.
    If the child is febrile, a complete examination to evaluate the fever is necessary.

LABORATORY TESTING

In the febrile child, a lumbar puncture should always be considered. Detection of clinical signs of meningitis depends on the individual physician's ability and training as well as the age of the child. If the physician has any doubt regarding the possibility of intracranial infection, the patient should have either an immediate lumbar puncture or empiric antibiotic treatment with emergency hospital transport. Other laboratory testing should be directed toward evaluation of the fever. With a first febrile seizure, serum electrolytes, calcium, magnesium, and phosphorus are not usually necessary. A blood glucose is indicated if the child has a prolonged postictal state. Neuroimaging or an electroencephalogram (EEG) is not needed.

In the **afebrile** child or the child with recurrent seizures the laboratory evaluation can include a complete blood count, electrolytes, calcium, magnesium, phosphorus, blood urea nitrogen, creatinine, glucose, liver function tests, and toxicologic screening. An electroencephalogram often demonstrates an abnormality, but a normal one does not rule out seizures. The diagnostic yield of the EEG can be increased by eye closure, photic stimulation, hyperventilation, or sleep deprivation. Magnetic resonance imaging is useful in evaluating children with complex partial seizures, a focal neurologic deficit, seizures of increasing frequency or severity, or resistance to medication and in evaluating all adolescents with a first seizure. Computed tomography scans are rarely helpful.

New evidence suggests that the long QT syndrome may be responsible for some cases of unexplained "seizures" or syncope. These children often present with "seizures" following emotional events or exercise. They may have a family history of sudden death or unexplained syncope. In these cases, an EKG should be done with the corrected QT interval (QT_c) calculated manually [$QT_c = QT_{(seconds)}$/square root RR interval (seconds)], as automated calculations may be misleading (Fig. 7.2).

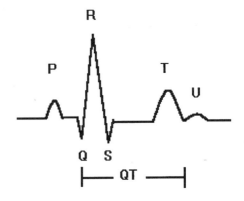

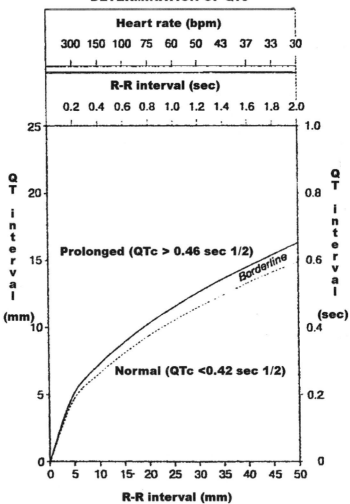

FIGURE 7.2. Determination of QTc. Adapted from Ackerman MJ. The long QT syndrome. *Pediatr Rev* 1998;19:236. Reproduced by permission of *Pediatrics in Review*.

Seizures in the newborn period may be due to infection, metabolic encephalopathy, or anoxic encephalopathy and require a complete evaluation. This usually requires hospitalization and specialty consultation.

DIAGNOSIS

The diagnosis of seizures is generally made based on the history and physical examination. Table 7.3 lists conditions commonly mistaken for seizures.

Febrile seizures are divided into simple febrile seizures, which are generalized and last less than 15 minutes, and complex febrile seizures, which last more than 15 minutes, are focal, or occur more than once in 24 hours.

For nonfebrile seizures multiple classification systems exist. Table 7.4 describes common seizure types.

Other syndromes in pediatric epilepsy have also been identified (Table 7.5).

T ABLE 7.3. Conditions mistaken for seizures in children

Breath-holding spells
Gastroesophageal reflux–induced apnea
Benign paroxysmal vertigo
Cough syncope
Prolonged QT syndrome
Night terrors
Rage attacks
Masturbation with rhythmic copulatory movements
Motor tics
Pseudo-seizures

Adapted from Haslam RH. Nonfebrile seizures. *Pediatr Rev* 1997;18:39.

T ABLE 7.4. Common seizure types*

Simple partial seizure	Focal tonic or clonic movements often of the head, lasting 20–30 seconds. Child remains conscious. EEG usually shows unilateral spikes or sharp waves in the anterior temporal region.
Complex partial seizure	May have an aura followed by repetitive stereotyped behaviors. Has a loss of consciousness by definition. EEG usually shows spikes or sharp waves in the anterior temporal or frontal region.
Simple absence seizures	Usually begin at 5 or 6 years of age. Loss of consciousness lasts for 5–20 seconds with no postictal period. EEG shows 2–2.5/sec or 3.5–4.5/sec generalized spike and wave discharges.
Primary generalized	Formerly called "grand mal." Sudden loss of consciousness
Tonic clonic seizures	Followed by intense muscle contraction (tonic) and or symmetric jerking movements (clonic). Patients have a postictal period with headache.

*Other syndromes in pediatric epilepsy have also been identified (see Table 7.5.).
Adapted from Haslam RH. Nonfebrile seizures. *Pediatr Rev* 1997;18:39.

T ABLE 7.5. Epileptic syndromes in children

Syndrome	Clinical Description	EEG Findings	Treatment	Prognosis
Infantile spasms	Onset between 4 and 8 months of age. Seizures consist of repetitive volleys of brief flexion or extension contractions of the neck, trunk, and extremities that persist for 10 to 30 seconds per volley. Frequently, loss of developmental milestones with the onset of seizures.	High-voltage bilaterally asynchronous, and irregular high-voltage spike and wave pattern.	Adrenocorticotropic hormone (ACTH) Benzodiazepines Vigabatrin (infantile spasms and tuberous sclerosis) Epilepsy surgery when focal onset	Guarded; majority have poor outcome with persistent seizures.
Lennox-Gastaut	Common in preschool children. A mixture of seizures, including myoclonic, generalized tonic-clonic, partial, absence, and atonic, is characteristic. Status epilepticus is frequent. Often occurs in children who previously had encephalopathy.	Abnormal background activity, slow spike-waves, and multifocal abnormalities.	Valproic acid Benzodiazepines Ketogenic diet	Unfavorable; high association with mental retardation and behavioral problems

	Clinical features	EEG	Treatment	Outcome
Landau-Kleffner	Average onset between 3 and 5 years of age; more common in boys. Loss of language (slow or rapid) in a previously healthy child. 70% have an associated seizure disorder as well as behavioral problems. Seizures may be focal or generalized tonic-clonic, atypical absence, and partial complex.	High-amplitude spike and wave discharges may be bitemporal, multifocal, or generalized. EEG changes always more apparent during non-REM sleep.	Valproic acid, Prednisone, Speech therapy, Subpial resection?	Variable; onset before 2 years of age has poor outcome. Most have significant speech dysfunctions as adults.
Benign childhood epilepsy with centrotemporal (rolandic) spikes	Peak onset between 9 and 10 years of age (range, 2 to 14 years). Majority occur during sleep. Child awakened by unilateral tonic-clonic contractions of the face, paresthesias of tongue and cheek, and occasional clonic seizures of ipsilateral upper extremity. Child is conscious but aphasic for several minutes.	Repetitive spike discharges confined to the centro-temporal area with normal background activity.	Occasional seizures require no therapy. Frequent seizures controlled by carbamazepine	Excellent; spontaneous remission by adolescence.
Juvenile myoclonic epilepsy (Janz syndrome)	Onset between 12 and 16 years of age. Myoclonic jerks on awakening that diminish later in day. Most develop early morning generalized tonic-clonic seizures.	A 4–6-per-second irregular spike and wave pattern enhanced by photic stimulation.	Valproic acid	Excellent, but valproic acid is required lifelong.

Used with permission from Haslam RH. Nonfebrile seizures. *Pediatr Rev* 1997;18:39.

MANAGEMENT

Febrile Seizure

Reassurance is the main management for a febrile seizure. These seizures do not cause brain damage. The seizure recurs in approximately one-third of patients. Recurrence risk is higher in younger children and those with a family history of febrile seizures. Fewer than 5% of children go on to develop epilepsy, with a higher risk found in children with preexisting abnormal development, family history of epilepsy, or complex febrile seizure. Vigorous control of subsequent fevers has not been shown to reduce the recurrence rate. Medications are rarely indicated.

Nonfebrile Seizures

Management of nonfebrile seizures is more problematic. Table 7.5 lists the management of the specific seizure syndromes. Absence seizures should be treated at diagnosis. If the child has a single tonic-clonic seizure, a normal EEG, and a negative family history, the risk of recurrence is low and antepileptics are usually not indicated. If the seizure recurs within a year, anticonvulsants are usually initiated. The medication is selected based on the seizure type as well as side effect profile, price, and dosing regimen (Table 7.6). Once the drug is initiated, the dose should be gradually increased until side effects are experienced or the maintenance dose is reached. If the child has a seizure while on the maintenance dose, the medication trial is considered a failure and a new medication is titrated up, while the first is tapered off. Serum levels are not used to determine dosing, and many patients tolerate levels above the recommended range. Levels are generally indicated to document the blood level when on a maintenance dose. They also may be useful when noncompliance is suspected, when the child is growing rapidly and may need a higher medication dose, when it is necessary to document a level at which the medication is not controlling seizures, or when disabled patients cannot report symptoms.

Medication interactions are common, especially with oral contraceptives, other anticonvulsants, and between carbamazepine (Tegretol) and erythromycin (E-Mycin, EES, Pediazole).

FOLLOW-UP

Patients who are on anticonvulsant therapy are seen approximately every 3 months, more frequently if seizures are not well controlled. Consideration may be given to anticonvulsant withdrawal if the child is seizure-free for 2 years and has a normal EEG. Withdrawal is best accomplished by gradually tapering off the medications. If the seizures recur, the medication is restarted. If the seizures recur following two trials off medication, lifelong therapy may be needed.

PATIENT EDUCATION

When a child has a seizure, he or she should be placed on a safe surface on his or her side or abdomen with face downward to reduce the risk of aspiration. Nothing should be placed in the mouth. If the seizure lasts more than 10 minutes, the child should be brought to the nearest medical facility. If the seizure resolved spontaneously, the physician should be notified of the event.

TABLE 7.6. Common anticonvulsant drugs

Drug	Seizure Type	Oral Dose	Therapeutic Serum Level		Side Effects and Toxicities
			µg/mL	µmol/L	
ACTH	Infantile spasms	20 U IM/24 h for 2 wk. If no response, increase to 30 U and then 40 U IM/24 h for an additional wk	—	—	Hyperglycemia, hypertension, electrolyte abnormalities, infections, sudden death
Carbamazepine (Tegretol)	Partial epilepsy Tonic-clonic	Begin 10 mg/kg per 24 h. Increase by 5 mg/kg per 24 h every wk to 20–30 mg/kg per 24 h in two or three divided doses	4–12	17–50	Dizziness, drowsiness, diplopia, liver dysfunction, anemia, leukopenia
Clonazepam (Klonopin)	Myoclonic Infantile spasms Absence	Begin 0.05 mg/kg per 24 h. Increase by 0.05 mg/kg per wk. Maximum, 0.2 mg/kg per 24 h in two or three divided doses	6.3–56.8	0.02–0.18	Drowsiness, irritability, drooling, behavioral abnormalities, depression
Ethosuximide	Absence Myoclonic	Begin 10–20 mg/kg per 24 h in two divided doses; may be increased to 50 mg/kg per 24 h	40–160	280–710	Drowsiness, nausea, rarely blood dyscrasias
Gabapentin (add-on therapy) (Neurontin)	Partial epilepsy Tonic-clonic	Begin 300 mg/24 h. Increase by 300 mg/24 h every 3–5 days. Maximum 900–1,200 mg/24 h in three equally divided doses	<2	<11.7	Somnolence, dizziness, ataxia, headache, tremor, vomiting, nystagmus, fatigue. Gabapentin is cleared by the kidney; few side effects.
Lamotrigine (add-on therapy)	Partial epilepsy Tonic-clonic Lennox-Gastaut	Begin 2 mg/kg per 24 h in two equal doses. Increase to maintenance dose of 5–15 mg/kg per 24 h. Lower doses begin 0.5 mg/kg per 24 h to maintenance of 1–5 mg/kg per 24 h if used with valproic acid	1–4	4–39	Severe skin rashes, especially when given in combination with valproic acid. Drowsiness, headache, blurred vision

continued

TABLE 7.6. Common anticonvulsant drugs *(continued)*

Drug	Seizure Type	Oral Dose	Therapeutic Serum Level µg/mL	Therapeutic Serum Level µmol/L	Side Effects and Toxicities
Phenobarbital (Donnatal)	Tonic-clonic, Partial epilepsy	3 to 5 mg/kg per 2 h in one or two divided doses	15–40	65–170	Hyperactivity, irritability, short attention span, temper tantrums, altered sleep pattern, Stevens-Johnson syndrome, depression of cognitive function
Phenytoin (Dilantin)	Partial epilepsy, Tonic-clonic	5 to 6 mg/kg per 24 h in two divided doses	10–20	40–80	Hirsutism, gum hypertrophy, ataxia, skin rash, Stevens-Johnson syndrome
Primidone	Tonic-clonic, Partial epilepsy, Myoclonic	Begin 50 mg/24 h in two divided doses. Gradually increase to 150 to 500 mg/24 h divided into three equal doses	5–12	25–55	Aggressive behavior and personality changes similar to those for phenobarbital
Sodium valproate (Depacon)	Tonic-clonic, Absence, Myoclonic, Partial epilepsy, Unclassified	Begin 10 mg/kg per 24 h. Increase by 5 to 10 mg/kg per wk. Usual dose, 20 to 60 mg/kg per 24 h in two to three divided doses	50–100	350–700	Weight gain, alopecia, tremor, hepatotoxicity
Vigabatrin (add-on therapy; not yet available in US)	Partial epilepsy, Infantile spasms (tuberous sclerosis)	Begin 30–40 mg/kg per 24 h. Increase by 10 mg/kg per wk. Maximum, 80–100 mg/kg per 24 h in two equal doses	1.4–14	10.8–108	Agitation, drowsiness, weight gain, dizziness, headache, ataxia

Used with permission from Haslam RH. Nonfebrile seizures. *Pediatr Rev* 1997;18:39.

REFERRAL

Specialist referral depends on the level of expertise of the individual physician. Seizures in the newborn period generally require referral, as their evaluation and management can be quite complex. If seizures are not controlled after trials of two or three medications, the child should generally be referred to an epileptic specialist, as seizure control is likely to be difficult and less common medications, surgery, the ketogenic diet, or a vagus nerve stimulator may be needed.

REFERENCES

Ackerman MJ. The long QT syndrome. *Pediatr Rev* 1998;19:232.

Haslam RH. Nonfebrile seizures. *Pediatr Rev* 1997;18:39.

Hirtz DG. Febrile seizures. *Pediatr Rev* 1997;18:5.

Marks WJ, Garcia PA. Management of seizures and epilepsy. *Am Fam Physician* 1998;57:1589.

Provisional Committee on Quality Improvement, Subcommittee on Febrile seizures. American Academy of Pediatrics. *Pediatrics* 1996;97:769.

Patient Education/Resources

Epilepsy Foundation. 800-EFA-1000. www.efa.org. Patient education, online bookstore, teen chat, summer camps.

APPENDIX

See Tables 7.7 and 7.8.

TABLE 7.7. Blood pressure levels for the 90th and 95th percentiles of blood pressure for boys age 1 to 17 years by percentiles of height

Age	*BP†	Systolic BP (mm Hg)							Diastolic BP (mm Hg)						
	Height Percentiles →	5%	10%	25%	50%	75%	90%	95%	5%	10%	25%	50%	75%	90%	95%
1	90th	94	95	97	98	100	102	102	50	51	52	53	54	54	55
	95th	98	99	101	102	104	106	106	55	55	56	57	58	59	59
2	90th	98	99	100	102	104	105	106	55	55	56	57	58	59	59
	95th	101	102	104	106	108	109	110	59	59	60	61	62	63	63
3	90th	100	101	103	105	107	108	109	59	59	60	61	62	63	63
	95th	104	105	107	109	111	112	113	63	63	64	65	66	67	67
4	90th	102	103	105	107	109	110	111	62	62	63	64	65	66	66
	95th	106	107	109	111	113	114	115	66	67	67	68	69	70	71
5	90th	104	105	106	108	110	112	112	65	65	66	67	68	69	69
	95th	108	109	110	112	114	115	116	69	70	70	71	72	73	74
6	90th	105	106	108	110	111	113	114	67	68	69	70	70	71	72
	95th	109	110	112	114	115	117	117	72	72	73	74	75	76	76
7	90th	106	107	109	111	113	114	115	69	70	71	72	72	73	74
	95th	110	111	113	115	116	118	119	74	74	75	76	77	78	78
8	90th	107	108	110	112	114	115	116	71	71	72	73	74	75	75
	95th	111	112	114	116	118	119	120	75	76	76	77	78	79	80

Age	BP Percentile†	Systolic BP by Height Percentile*							Diastolic BP by Height Percentile*						
9	90th	109	110	112	113	115	117	117	72	73	73	74	75	76	77
	95th	113	114	116	117	119	121	121	76	77	78	79	80	80	81
10	90th	110	112	113	115	117	118	119	73	74	74	75	76	77	78
	95th	114	115	117	119	121	122	123	77	78	79	80	80	81	82
11	90th	112	113	115	117	119	120	121	74	74	75	76	77	78	78
	95th	116	117	119	121	123	124	125	78	79	79	80	81	82	83
12	90th	115	116	117	119	121	123	123	75	75	76	77	78	78	79
	95th	119	120	121	123	125	126	127	79	79	80	81	82	83	83
13	90th	117	118	120	122	124	125	126	75	76	76	77	78	79	80
	95th	121	122	124	126	128	129	130	79	80	81	82	83	83	84
14	90th	120	121	123	125	126	128	128	76	76	77	78	79	80	80
	95th	124	125	127	128	130	132	132	80	81	81	82	83	84	85
15	90th	123	124	125	127	129	131	131	77	77	78	79	80	81	81
	95th	127	128	129	131	133	134	135	81	82	83	83	84	85	86
16	90th	125	126	128	130	132	133	134	79	80	80	81	82	82	83
	95th	129	130	132	134	136	137	138	83	83	84	85	86	87	87
17	90th	128	129	131	133	134	136	136	81	81	82	83	84	85	85
	95th	132	133	135	136	138	140	140	85	85	86	87	88	89	89

*Height percentile determined by standard growth curves.

†Blood pressure percentile determined by a single measurement.

Used with permission of the American Academy of Pediatrics. Natural high blood pressure education working group in hypertension control in children and adolescents. Updates in the 1987 task force report on high blood pressure in children and adolescents. Pediatrics 1996;98(4).

T ABLE 7.8. Blood pressure levels for the 90th and 95th percentiles of blood pressure for girls age 1 to 17 years by percentiles of height

Age	Height Percentiles → *BP† →	Systolic BP (mm Hg)							Diastolic BP (mm Hg)						
		5%	10%	25%	50%	75%	90%	95%	5%	10%	25%	50%	75%	90%	95%
1	90th	97	98	99	100	102	103	104	53	53	53	54	55	56	56
	95th	101	102	103	104	105	107	107	57	57	57	58	59	60	60
2	90th	99	99	100	102	103	104	105	57	57	58	58	59	60	61
	95th	102	103	104	105	107	108	109	61	61	62	62	63	64	65
3	90th	100	100	102	103	104	105	106	61	61	61	62	63	63	64
	95th	104	104	105	107	108	109	110	65	65	65	66	67	67	68
4	90th	101	102	103	104	106	107	108	63	63	64	65	65	66	67
	95th	105	106	107	108	109	111	111	67	67	68	69	69	70	71
5	90th	103	103	104	106	107	108	109	65	66	66	67	68	68	69
	95th	107	107	108	110	111	112	113	69	70	70	71	72	72	73
6	90th	104	105	106	107	109	110	111	67	67	68	69	69	70	71
	95th	108	109	110	111	112	114	114	71	71	72	73	73	74	75
7	90th	106	107	108	109	110	112	112	69	69	69	70	71	72	72
	95th	110	110	112	113	114	115	116	73	73	73	74	75	76	76
8	90th	108	109	110	111	112	113	114	70	70	71	71	72	73	74
	95th	112	112	113	115	116	117	118	74	74	75	75	76	77	78

Age	BP percentile†	Systolic BP by height percentile*							Diastolic BP by height percentile*						
9	90th	110	110	112	113	114	115	116	71	72	72	73	74	74	75
	95th	114	114	115	117	118	119	120	75	76	76	77	78	78	79
10	90th	112	112	114	115	116	117	118	73	73	73	74	75	76	76
	95th	116	116	117	119	120	121	122	77	77	77	78	79	80	80
11	90th	114	114	116	117	118	119	120	74	74	74	75	76	77	77
	95th	118	118	119	121	122	123	124	78	78	78	79	80	81	81
12	90th	116	116	118	119	120	121	122	75	75	75	76	77	78	78
	95th	120	120	121	123	124	125	126	79	79	79	80	81	82	82
13	90th	118	118	119	121	122	123	124	76	76	76	78	78	79	80
	95th	121	122	123	125	126	127	128	80	80	80	82	82	83	84
14	90th	119	120	121	122	124	125	126	77	77	78	79	79	80	81
	95th	123	124	125	126	128	129	130	81	81	82	83	83	84	85
15	90th	121	121	122	124	125	126	127	78	78	79	79	80	81	82
	95th	124	125	126	128	129	130	131	82	82	83	83	84	85	86
16	90th	122	122	123	125	126	127	128	79	79	79	80	81	82	82
	95th	125	126	127	128	130	131	132	83	83	83	84	85	86	86
17	90th	122	123	124	125	126	128	128	79	79	79	80	81	82	82
	95th	126	126	127	129	130	131	132	83	83	83	84	85	86	86

* Height percentile determined by standard growth curves.

† Blood pressure percentile determined by a single measurement.

Used with permission of the American Academy of Pediatrics. Natural high blood pressure education working group in hypertension control in children and adolescents. Updates in the 1987 task force report on high blood pressure in children and adolescents. Pediatrics 1996;98(4).

CHAPTER 8

Chronic Conditions

Asthma

Asthma is the most common chronic disease in childhood, affecting 4% to 5% of all children. Despite advances in understanding the pathophysiology of the disease, over the past 20 years the number of affected children and the number of mortalities secondary to asthma have increased dramatically. Ideal management continues to hinge on the ongoing therapeutic relationship between the child, family, and physician.

HISTORY OF PRESENT ILLNESS

The history should include the presence of shortness of breath, wheezing, or cough. Does the child have retractions? Are these symptoms constant or only present with upper respiratory infection? When was the first time the symptoms appeared? Ask whether the child or caregivers have noticed exacerbating factors such as allergen exposure (pets, dust, pollen), level of air pollution, cold air exposure, exercise, or emotional stress. Do the symptoms vary with the season (seasonal pollens) or time of day (early-morning symptoms are associated with a poorer prognosis)? Is the child exposed to irritants such as cigarette smoke or wood or kerosene heat?

PAST MEDICAL HISTORY

Asthma is more common in children who were premature or had bronchopulmonary dysplasia. In the child with a known history of asthma, has there been any previous use of corticosteroids, hospitalizations, life-threatening episodes, or intubations? Which medications has the child used?

FAMILY HISTORY

Do others in the family have asthma, allergy, nasal polyps, or cystic fibrosis?

SOCIAL HISTORY

Who lives with the child? What resources are available to cope with this chronic illness? Are parents missing work because of the child's illness? Has the child's behavior changed since these symptoms began?

PHYSICAL EXAMINATION

Areas of particular emphasis on physical exam include the following:

Chest: hyperexpansion, use of accessory muscles

Lungs: wheezing, including forced expiration, prolonged expiration

Nose: nasal polyps, nasal secretions, mucosa

Skin: atopic dermatitis, eczema

LABORATORY TESTING

Laboratory testing is not generally needed specifically for the diagnosis of asthma. If nasal polyps or other symptoms of cystic fibrosis are present, a sweat test may be needed. Spirometry or pulmonary function testing may be useful for confirmation of the diagnosis or for follow-up. Skin testing or *in vitro* assays (radioallergosorbent test [RAST]) may be used to identify specific allergens, especially if asthma is difficult to control or the family is reluctant to take measures to control home allergens.

DIAGNOSIS

Children with asthma present in a variety of ways. Some have classic symptoms of wheezing or shortness of breath, especially with upper respiratory infection or allergen exposure. Others have nighttime cough or shortness of breath with exercise. The diagnosis requires a history consistent with asthma, evidence of at least partially reversible airflow obstruction (usually obtained with a peak flow meter; see later), and no evidence of another cause. Table 8.1 lists differential diagnostic considerations. As asthma is very common in children, specific evaluation to rule out other causes is only performed when indicated by the history, physical examination, or clinical course.

T ABLE 8.1.   Differential diagnosis of asthma in children

Allergic rhinitis and sinusitis
Foreign body in the respiratory tree
Gastroesophageal reflux with aspiration
Laryngotracheomalacia, tracheal stenosis, bronchostenosis
Cystic fibrosis
Heart disease

From National Asthma Education and Prevention Program, National Heart, Lung and Blood Institute. Expert Panel Report 2. Clinical practice guidelines for the diagnosis and management of asthma. Bethesda, NIH Pub No. 97-4051, April 1997.

MONITORING

Peak flow monitoring is essential for asthma management. Children older than 5 or 6 years of age are usually able to use peak flow meters. Home peak flow monitors generally cost less than $40 and may be covered by third-party payers. Patients with moderate asthma should measure their peak flow approximately twice daily, and all patients should do them whenever they have symptoms. These readings are recorded in a diary that is brought to office visits (Fig. 8.1). Table 8.2 lists predicted peak flow measurements based on age and height. Over time, patients can determine their own personal best, keeping in mind that this should increase as the child grows.

MANAGEMENT

Management is based on disease severity as defined in Table 8.3. All patients are prescribed a beta agonist for use when symptoms are present. Antiinflammatory medications are added based on the disease severity (Table 8.4 and Figure 8.2). Rapid symptom control can be attained by initiating medication for a higher severity than the expected baseline. Once symptoms are controlled, the medication can be reduced to maintenance levels. Keeping in mind the caregiver's literacy, written instructions and charts can clarify complicated regimens (see later). With the recent demonstration of improved long-term pulmonary function with early initiation of antiinflammatory medications, these should be added as recommended, and continued even after symptoms are controlled. Table 8.5 lists common medications used for asthma management.

EXACERBATIONS

The peak flow should be measured whenever the child has increased symptoms. These readings can be classified as green zone (80% to 100% of predicted), yellow zone (50% to 79% of predicted), and red zone (less than 50%) (Fig. 8.1). Caregivers should be instructed in individualized management of the child if the reading is in the yellow or red zone (Fig. 8.3). Generally, this instruction takes the form of an individualized asthma action plan. The plan includes dosing for beta agonists, guidelines for increasing inhaled steroids or for adding oral steroids, and recommendations for when to call the physician or ambulance (Fig. 8.4). Patients may need to be given a prescription for oral steroids before the exacerbation, so that the steroids are available when needed.

Many patients are seen in the office for an asthmatic exacerbation. The office staff should be trained to recognize the severe acute asthmatic attack and initiate immediate treatment. Initial assessment includes a brief history and physical examination, including measurement of respiratory and heart rate, peak flow (except in severe exacerbations) auscultation of the lungs, and observation for accessory muscle use. If pulse oximetry and supplemental oxygen are available, the oxygen saturation should be measured and supplemental oxygen should be used to maintain oxygen saturation at greater than 90%. An inhaled beta agonist should be given immediately, with a metered dose inhaler or nebulizer. These treatments may be repeated every 20 minutes for a mild exacerbation or given continuously for a severe one. Ipatropium bromide may be added to the beta agonist to augment the effect. After the treatments are given, the child should have serial reassessments. The decision for hospital admission takes into account the severity of the attack, the child's response to treatment, the likely cause of the exacerbation, and caregiver capabilities. Table 8.6 outlines criteria for hospital admission.

How To Use Your Peak Flow Meter

A peak flow meter helps you check how well your asthma is controlled. Peak flow meters are most helpful for people with moderate or severe asthma.

This guide will tell you (1) how to find your personal best peak flow number, (2) how to use your personal best number to set your peak flow zones, (3) how to take your peak flow, and (4) when to take your peak flow to check your asthma each day.

Starting Out: Find Your Personal Best Peak Flow Number

To find your personal best peak flow number, take your peak flow each day for 2 to 3 weeks. Your asthma should be under good control during this time. Take your peak flow as close to the times listed below as you can. (These times for taking your peak flow are only for finding your personal best peak flow. To check your asthma

each day, you will take your peak flow in the morning. This is discussed on the next page.)

- Between noon and 2:00 p.m. each day.

- Each time you take your quick-relief medicine to relieve symptoms. (Measure your peak flow after you take your medicine.)

- Any other time your doctor suggests.

Write down the number you get for each peak flow reading. The highest peak flow number you had during the 2 to 3 weeks is your personal best.

Your personal best can change over time. Ask your doctor when to check for a new personal best.

Your Peak Flow Zones

Your peak flow zones are based on your personal best peak flow number. The zones will help you check your asthma and take the right actions to keep it controlled. The colors used with each zone come from the traffic light.

Green Zone (80 to 100 percent of your personal best) signals **good control**. Take your usual daily long-term-control medicines, if you take any. Keep taking these medicines even when you are in the yellow or red zones.

Yellow Zone (50 to 79 percent of your personal best) signals caution: **your asthma is getting worse**. Add quick-relief medicines. You might need to increase other asthma medicines as directed by your doctor.

Red Zone (below 50 percent of your personal best) signals **medical alert!** Add or increase quick-relief medicines and call your doctor now.

Ask your doctor to write an action plan for you that tells you:

- The peak flow numbers for your green, yellow, and red zones. Mark the zones on your peak flow meter with colored tape or a marker.

- The medicines you should take while in each peak flow zone.

FIGURE 8.1. How to use your peak flow meter. (U.S. Department of Health and Human Services, National Institutes of Health. Practical guide for the diagnosis and management of asthma. NIH Publication no. 97-4053. Bethesda, MD: NIH.)

How To Take Your Peak Flow

1. Move the marker to the bottom of the numbered scale.

2. Stand up or sit up straight.

3. Take a deep breath. Fill your lungs all the way.

4. Hold your breath while you place the mouthpiece in your mouth, between your teeth. Close your lips around it. Do **not** put your tongue inside the hole.

5. Blow out as hard and fast as you can. Your peak flow meter will measure how fast you can blow out air.

6. Write down the number you get. But if you cough or make a mistake, do not write down the number. Do it over again.

7. Repeat steps 1 through 6 two more times. Write down the highest of the three numbers. This is your peak flow number.

8. Check to see which peak flow <u>zone</u> your peak flow number is in. Do the actions your doctor told you to do while in that zone.

Your doctor may ask you to write down your peak flow numbers each day. You can do this on a calendar or other paper. This will help you and your doctor see how your asthma is doing over time.

FIGURE 8.1.   *continued*

Checking Your Asthma: When To Use Your Peak Flow Meter

- **Every morning** when you wake up, *before* you take medicine. **Make this part of** your daily routine.

- **When you are having asthma symptoms or an attack.** And after taking medicine for the attack. This can tell you how bad your asthma attack is and whether your medicine is working.

- Any other time your doctor suggests.

If you use more than one peak flow meter (such as at home and at school), be sure that both meters are the same brand.

Bring to Each of Your Doctor's Visits:

- Your peak flow meter.

- Your peak flow numbers if you have written them down each day.

Also, ask your doctor or nurse to check how you use your peak flow meter—just to be sure you are doing it right.

FIGURE 8.1. *continued*

T ABLE 8.2. Predicted average peak expiratory flow rates for normal children

Height (in.)	PEFR (L/min)	Height (in.)	PEFR (L/min)
43	147	56	320
44	160	57	334
45	173	58	347
46	187	59	360
47	200	60	373
48	214	61	387
49	227	62	400
50	240	63	413
51	254	64	427
52	267	65	440
53	280	66	454
54	293	67	467
55	307		

From Barone MA, ed. Harriet Lane Handbook, 14th ed. St. Louis: Mosby, 1971.
PEFR, peak expiratory flow rate.

T ABLE 8.3. Classification of severity of chronic asthma[a]

Classification	Days with symptoms	Nights with symptoms	PEF (% best)[b] FEV$_1$ (% predicted)[c]	PEF variability[b]
Mild intermittent	≤2/wk	≤2/mo	≥80%	<20%
Mild persistent	>2/wk	3–4/mo	≥80%	20–30%
Moderate persistent	Daily Daily adrenergic inhaler	≥1/wk	>60% but <80%	>30%
Severe persistent	Continual Limited activity Frequent exacerbations[c]	Frequent	≤60%	>30%

FEV$_1$, forced expiratory volume over 1 second; PEF, peak expiratory flow.
[a]The features of a given patient's severity are highly variable and may overlap severity grades. The presence of any one feature of a severity grade is sufficient to place a child in that severity category.
[b]For children older than 5 years who can use a spirometer or peak flowmeter.
[c]Patients at any severity level can experience mild, moderate, or severe exacerbations. An exacerbation is defined as an increase in symptoms lasting hours to days and requiring additonal emergency medications.
From Eggleston PA. Asthma. In: McMillan JA, DeAngelis CD, Feigin RD, Warshaw JB, eds. *Oski's pediatrics: principles and practice.* New York: Lippincott Williams and Wilkins, 1999.

T ABLE 8.4. Recommended chronic medications for different severity levels of chronic disease

Severity level	Symptomatic medication	Controller medication
Mild intermittent	Short-acting adrenergic agent	None
Mild persistent	Short-acting adrenergic agonist	Cromolyn, nedocromil *or* Low-dose inhaled steroids *or* Leukotriene modifiers
Moderate persistent	Short-acting adrenergic agonist	Moderate-dose inhaled steroids *or* Low-dose inhaled steroids *and* Leukotriene modifiers Theophylline Long-acting adrenergic agonist
Severe persistent	Short-acting adrenergic agonist	High-dose inhaled steroids *and* Theophylline Long-acting adrenergic agonist

From Eggleston PA. Asthma. In: McMillan JA, DeAngelis CD, Feigin RD, Warshaw JB, eds. *Oski's pediatrics: principles and practice.* New York: Lippincott Williams & Wilkins, 1999.

Hospitalization should also be considered if the child has had a severe exacerbation in the past or if the peak flow stays less than 70% of predicted. For home management, oral steroids for a 3- to 5-day course are generally needed, though in mild exacerbations high-dose inhaled steroids may be effective. Caregivers should be aware of the method to reach the physician, including after hours, and the method to activate the emergency medical system. Allergen and irritant exposure should be minimized (see later).

EXERCISE-INDUCED ASTHMA

When asthma symptoms are present only with exercise, the patient may be treated with a beta agonist, two to four puffs immediately before exercise. Cromolyn (Intal) or nedocromil (Tilade) are also effective. If a longer duration of action is needed, a long-acting beta agonist (salmetrol, [Serevent]) may be used at least 30 minutes before exercise. Patients and parents should be reassured that asthma does not preclude participation in athletics, even at the professional level.

MEDICATION DELIVERY

Medications are generally delivered by metered dose inhaler (MDI) (Fig. 8.5). A spacer added to a MDI allows more of the medication to be delivered to the lungs instead of the throat. Inhaled steroids should always be dosed with a spacer and patients should rinse and spit after use. Breath-actuated devices are becoming available and may be easier to use. Dry powder inhalers have the advantage of not requiring fluorocarbon propellants and can be used consistently in children more than 5 years of age. Nebulizers

Stepwise Approach for Managing Infants and Young Children (5 Years of Age and Younger) With Acute or Chronic Asthma Symptoms

Long-Term Control

Step 4
Severe
Persistent

- Daily anti-inflammatory medication
  - High-dose inhaled steroid* with spacer and face mask
  - If needed, add oral steroids (2 mg/kg/day); reduce to lowest daily or alternate-day dose that stabilizes symptoms

Step 3
Moderate
Persistent

- Daily anti-inflammatory medication. Either:
  - Medium-dose inhaled steroid* with spacer and face mask
  Once control is established, consider:
  - Lower medium-dose inhaled steroid* with spacer and face mask and nedocromil (1-2 puffs bid-qid)
  OR
  - Lower medium-dose inhaled steroid* with spacer and face mask and theophylline (10 mg/kg/day up to 16 mg/kg/day for children ≥1 year of age, to a serum concentration of 5-15 mcg/mL)**

Step 2
Mild
Persistent

- Daily anti-inflammatory medication.
  - Infants and young children usually begin with a trial of cromolyn (nebulizer is preferred—1 ampule tid-qid; or MDI—1-2 puffs tid-qid) or nedocromil (MDI only—1-2 puffs bid-qid)
  OR
  - Low-dose inhaled steroid* with spacer and face mask

Step 1
Mild
Intermittent

- No daily medication needed.

Quick-Relief	
All Patients	Bronchodilator as needed for symptoms: Short-acting inhaled beta$_2$-agonist by nebulizer (0.05 mg/kg in 2-3 cc of saline) or inhaler with face mask and spacer (2-4 puffs; for exacerbations, repeat q 20 minutes for up to 1 hour) or oral beta$_2$-agonist.

With viral respiratory infection, use short-acting inhaled beta$_2$-agonist q 4 to 6 hours up to 24 hours (longer with physician consult) but, in general, if repeated more than once every 6 weeks, consider moving to next step up. Consider oral steroids if the exacerbation is moderate to severe or at the onset of the infection if the patient has a history of severe exacerbations. |

* See Estimated Comparative Dosages for Inhaled Steroids on page 38.

** For children <1 year of age: usual max mg/kg/day = 0.2 (age in weeks) + 5.

NOTES:

■ *The stepwise approach presents general guidelines to assist clinical decisionmaking. Asthma is highly variable; clinicians should tailor medication plans to the needs of individual patients.*

■ **Gain control** as quickly as possible. Either start with aggressive therapy (e.g., *add* a course of oral steroids or a higher dose of inhaled steroids to the therapy that corresponds to the patient's initial step of severity); or start at the step that corresponds to the patient's initial severity and step up treatment, if necessary.

■ **Step down.** Review treatment every 1 to 6 months. If control is sustained for at least 3 months, a gradual stepwise reduction in treatment may be possible.

■ **Step up.** If control is not achieved, consider step up. Inadequate control is indicated by increased use of short-acting beta$_2$-agonists and in: step 1 when patient uses a short-acting beta$_2$-agonist more than two times a week; steps 2 and 3 when patient uses short-acting beta$_2$-agonist on a daily basis OR more than three to four times a day. But before stepping up: review patient inhaler technique, compliance, and environmental control (avoidance of allergens or other precipitant factors).

■ A course of oral steroids (prednisolone) may be needed at any time and step.

■ Referral to an asthma specialist for consultation or comanagement is *recommended* for patients requiring step 3 or 4 care. Referral may be *considered* for step 2 care.

■ For a list of brand names, see glossary.

FIGURE 8.2. Stepwise approach for managing infants and young children (5 years of age and younger) with acute or chronic asthma symptoms. (U.S. Department of Health and Human Services, National Institutes of Health. Practical guide for the diagnosis and management of asthma. NIH Publication No. 97-4053. Bethesda, MD: NIH.)

Management of Asthma Exacerbations: Home Treatment

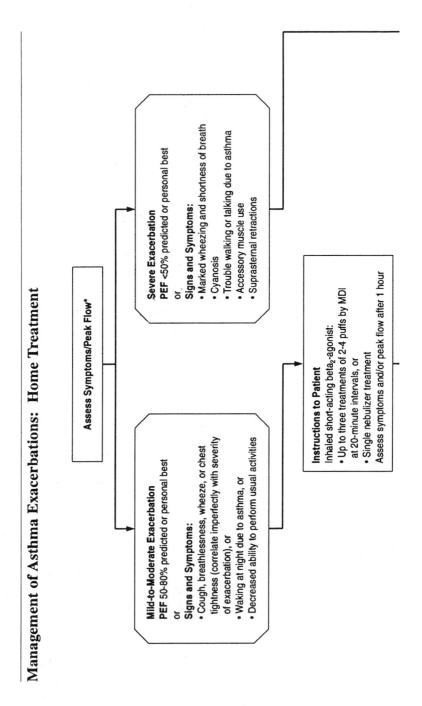

Assess Symptoms/Peak Flow*

Mild-to-Moderate Exacerbation
PEF 50-80% predicted or personal best
or
Signs and Symptoms:
• Cough, breathlessness, wheeze, or chest tightness (correlate imperfectly with severity of exacerbation), or
• Waking at night due to asthma, or
• Decreased ability to perform usual activities

Severe Exacerbation
PEF <50% predicted or personal best
or
Signs and Symptoms:
• Marked wheezing and shortness of breath
• Cyanosis
• Trouble walking or talking due to asthma
• Accessory muscle use
• Suprasternal retractions

Instructions to Patient
Inhaled short-acting beta$_2$-agonist:
• Up to three treatments of 2-4 puffs by MDI at 20-minute intervals, or
• Single nebulizer treatment
Assess symptoms and/or peak flow after 1 hour

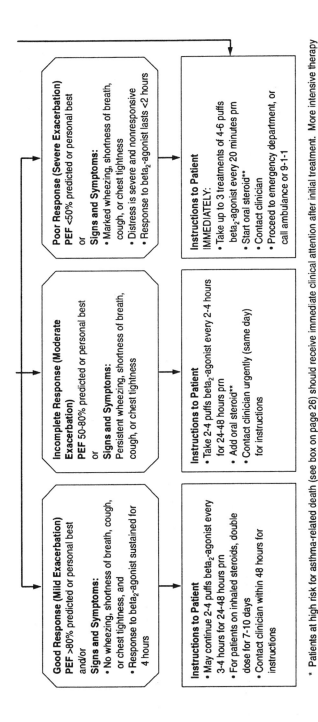

Good Response (Mild Exacerbation)
PEF >80% predicted or personal best
and/or
Signs and Symptoms:
- No wheezing, shortness of breath, cough, or chest tightness, and
- Response to beta$_2$-agonist sustained for 4 hours

Instructions to Patient
- May continue 2-4 puffs beta$_2$-agonist every 3-4 hours for 24-48 hours prn
- For patients on inhaled steroids, double dose for 7-10 days
- Contact clinician within 48 hours for instructions

Incomplete Response (Moderate Exacerbation)
PEF 50-80% predicted or personal best
or
Signs and Symptoms:
Persistent wheezing, shortness of breath, cough, or chest tightness

Instructions to Patient
- Take 2-4 puffs beta$_2$-agonist every 2-4 hours for 24-48 hours prn
- Add oral steroid**
- Contact clinician urgently (same day) for instructions

Poor Response (Severe Exacerbation)
PEF <50% predicted or personal best
or
Signs and Symptoms:
- Marked wheezing, shortness of breath, cough, or chest tightness
- Distress is severe and nonresponsive
- Response to beta$_2$-agonist lasts <2 hours

Instructions to Patient
IMMEDIATELY:
- Take up to 3 treatments of 4-6 puffs beta$_2$-agonist every 20 minutes prn
- Start oral steroid**
- Contact clinician
- Proceed to emergency department, or call ambulance or 9-1-1

* Patients at high risk for asthma-related death (see box on page 26) should receive immediate clinical attention after initial treatment. More intensive therapy may be required.
** Oral steroid dosages:
  Adult: 40-60 mg, single or 2 divided doses for 3-10 days.
  Child: 1-2 mg/kg/day, maximum 60 mg/day, for 3-10 days

FIGURE 8.3. Management of asthma exacerbations: home treatment. (U.S. Department of Health and Human Services, National Institutes of Health. Practical Guide for the Diagnosis and Management of Asthma. NIH Publication No. 97-4053. Bethesda, MD: NIH.)

T ABLE 8.5. Asthma medications

Medication	Age >12 years	Child <12 years	Comments
Inhaled Steroids			
Beclomethasone (Beclovent, Vanceril) (Use ½ no. of puffs for Vanceril double strength)	Low dose 8 puffs/day Medium dose 16 puffs/day High dose >20 puffs/day	4 puffs/day 12 puffs/day >16 puffs/day	(These apply to all the inhaled steroids.) Rinse mouth and spit after use Always use with a spacer Monitor growth Most effective antiinflammatory
Budesonide DPI (Pulmicort)	Low 1–2 inhalations/day Medium 2–3 inhalations/day High >3 inhalations/day	1–2 inhalations/days >2 inhalations/day	Use with a spacer with a face mask for young children.
Flunisolide (Aerobid)	Low 2–4 puffs/day Medium 4–8 puffs/day High >8 puffs/day	2–3 puffs/day 4–5 puffs/day >5 puffs/day	May be given once or twice daily
Fluticasone MDI (Flovent)	Low 2 puffs 110 μg/day Medium 2–6 puffs 110 μg/day High >3 puffs 220 μg/day	2–3 puffs 44 μg/day 2–4 puffs 110 μg/day >2 puffs 220 μg/day	
Fluticasone DPI (Flovent)	Low 2–6 inhalations 50 μg/day Medium 3–6 inhalations 100 μg/day High >2 inhalations 250 μg/day	2–4 inhalations (50 μg/day) 2–4 inhalations (100 μg/day) >2 inhalations (250 μg/day)	
Triamcinolone (Azmacort)	Low 6 puffs/day Medium 16 puffs/day High >20 puffs/day	5 puffs/day 10 puffs/day >12 puffs/day	
Oral Steroids			
Prednisone Tablets or suspension 5 mg/5 mL	40–60 mg/day for 3–10-day burst	1–2 mg/kg/day for 3–10-day burst	Continue burst until peak flow reaches 80% of personal best or symptoms resolve. Tapering has not been shown to prevent relapse.

Medication	Dose	Dose	Comments
Prednisolone Tablets or Pediapred 5 mg/5 mL	40–60 mg/day for 3–10-day burst	1–2 mg/kg/day for 3–10-day burst	
Anticholinergics			
Ipratropium bromide (Atrovent)	4–8 puffs as needed	4–8 puffs as needed	Used in acute exacerbations in combination with B₂ agonist
Nebulizer solution 0.5 mg/2.5 mL	Nebulizer: 0.5 mg every 30 minutes for 3 doses, then every 2–4 hours	Nebulizer: 0.25 mg every 20 minutes for 3 doses, then every 2–4 hours	May mix with albuterol in nebulizer; Not first-line therapy
Beta₂ Agonists			
Albuterol (Proventil, Ventolin)	2–4 puffs as needed	2–4 puffs as needed	Frequency of dosing depends on severity of symptoms
Nebulizer solution 5 mg/mL	Nebulizer: 2.5 mg	Nebulizer: 0.15 mg/kg or 1.25–2.5 mg/dose	Dose may be increased with severe exacerbations; May be diluted with cromolyn or ipratropium nebulizer solution for convenience; May cause tachycardia
Prediluted 2.5 mg/3 mL normal saline			
Pirbuterol (Maxair autohaler)	2 puffs every 4–6 hours		Not indicated for <12-year-olds; Breath actuated; Not studied for acute exacerbations
Long-Acting B₂ Agonist			
Salmeterol MDI (Serevent)	2 puffs every 12 hours		DPI approved for ages 4 and up; Not for acute exacerbation; Always use in conjunction with inhaled steroids

continued

TABLE 8.5. Asthma medications *(continued)*

Medication	Age >12 years	Child <12 years	Comments
Salmeterol DPI	One inhalation every 2 hours		Increased doses are not recommended
			May be used 30 minutes before exercise in exercise-induced asthma
Mast Cell Stabilizers			
Cromolyn (Intal)	2–4 puffs 3–4 times per day	1–2 puffs 3–4 times per day	Used first line in young children with mild to moderate persistent asthma
Nebulizer solution 10 mg/mL (2 mL vial)		Nebulizer 20 mg 4 times per day	Not effective if initiated less than 4 times per day
			Benefits seen in 4 weeks
			May decrease frequency to 3 times per day once symptoms are controlled
			Strong safety profile
			Can be combined with albuterol in the nebulizer after symptoms are controlled
			Nebulizer form preferred for young children
Nedocromil (Tilade)	2–4 puffs 2–3 times per day		Not indicated under age 12
			Benefit usually seen in 2 weeks
			Begin 4 times per day and decrease frequency once symptoms controlled
			Strong safety profile

Medication	Adult Dose	Child Dose	Comments
Leukotriene Modifier			
Zafirlukast (Accolate)	20 mg twice daily		Take 1 hour before or 2 hours after meals Not yet indicated for those under 12 years old
Montelukast (Singulair)	10 mg daily	5 mg daily	Use child dose for ages 6–14 Tablet taken in the evening without regard for food
Theophylline			
Theo 24, Theo-Dur, Slo-Bid	Start at 10 mg/kg/day Usual maximum dose 800 mg/day	Start at 10 mg/kg/day Usual maximum >1 year of age 16 mg/kg/day	Especially useful for nighttime symptoms Good serum concentration 5–15 mg/mL Monitoring of serum concentration is important as therapeutic dosages vary Multiple drug interactions Avoid alcohol-containing elixirs
Solution 80 mg/15 mL			

Abbreviations: MDI, metered-dose inhaler; DPI, dry powder inhaler.

Reference: National Asthma Education and Prevention Program, National Heart, Lung and Blood Institute. Expert Panel Report 2. Practical guide for the diagnosis and management of asthma. Bethesda, NIH Pub No. 97-4053, October 1997.

ASTHMA ACTION PLAN FOR _____

Doctor's Name _____ Date _____

Doctor's Phone Number _____

Hospital/Emergency Room Phone Number _____

Take These Long-Term-Control Medicines Each Day (include an anti-inflammatory)

GREEN ZONE: Doing Well

- No cough, wheeze, chest tightness, or shortness of breath during the day or night
- Can do usual activities

And, If a peak flow meter is used,
Peak flow: more than _____
(80% or more of my best peak flow)

My best peak flow is: _____

Before exercise

Medicine	How much to take	When to take it
	☐ 2 or ☐ 4 puffs	5 to 60 minutes before exercise

YELLOW ZONE: Asthma Is Getting Worse

- Cough, wheeze, chest tightness, or shortness of breath, or
- Waking at night due to asthma, or
- Can do some, but not all, usual activities

-Or-

Peak flow: _____ to _____
(50% - 80% of my best peak flow)

FIRST → Add: Quick-Relief Medicine – and keep taking your GREEN ZONE medicine

_____ ☐ 2 or ☐ 4 puffs, every 20 minutes for up to 1 hour
(short-acting beta₂-agonist) ☐ Nebulizer, once

SECOND → If your symptoms (and peak flow, if used) *return to GREEN ZONE* after 1 hour of above treatment:

☐ Take the quick-relief medicine every 4 hours for 1 to 2 days.
☐ Double the dose of your inhaled steroid for _____ (7-10) days.

-Or-

If your symptoms (and peak flow, if used) *do not return to GREEN ZONE* after 1 hour of above treatment:

☐ Take: _____ ☐ 2 or ☐ 4 puffs or ☐ Nebulizer
(short-acting beta₂-agonist)

☐ Add: _____ _____ mg. per day For _____ (3-10) days
(oral steroid)

☐ Call the doctor ☐ before/ ☐ within _____ hours after taking the oral steroid.

FIGURE 8.4. Asthmatic action plan. (U.S. Department of Health and Human Services, National Institutes of Health. Practical guide for the diagnosis and management of asthma. NIH Publication No. 97-4053. Bethesda, MD: NIH.)

RED ZONE: Medical Alert!

- Very short of breath, or
- Quick-relief medicines have not helped, or
- Cannot do usual activities, or
- Symptoms are same or get worse after 24 hours in Yellow Zone

-Or-

Peak flow: less than_____
(50% of my best peak flow)

Take this medicine:

❑ _____ ❑ 4 or ❑ 6 puffs or ❑ Nebulizer
(short-acting beta₂-agonist)

❑ _____ _____ mg.
(oral steroid)

Then call your doctor NOW. Go to the hospital or call for an ambulance if:
- You are still in the red zone after 15 minutes AND
- You have not reached your doctor.

⇨ ■ Take ❑ 4 or ❑ 6 puffs of your quick-relief medicine *AND*
■ Go to the hospital or call for an ambulance (_____) *NOW!*

DANGER SIGNS
- Trouble walking and talking due to shortness of breath
- Lips or fingernails are blue

FIGURE 8.4. *continued*

TABLE 8.6. Criteria for hospital admission for asthmatic exacerbation

Peak flow less than 50% of predicted following beta agonist treatments
Oxygen saturation less than 90% after beta agonist treatments
Drowsiness or confusion
Unreliable caregiver

HOW TO USE YOUR METERED-DOSE INHALER THE RIGHT WAY

Using an inhaler seems simple, but most patients do not use it the right way. When you use your inhaler the wrong way, less medicine gets to your lungs. (Your doctor may give you other types of inhalers.)

For the next 2 weeks, read these steps aloud as you do them or ask someone to read them to you. Ask your doctor or nurse to check how well you are using your inhaler.

Use your inhaler in one of the three ways pictured below (A or B are best, but C can be used if you have trouble with A and B).

Steps for Using Your Inhaler

Getting ready

1. Take off the cap and shake the inhaler.
2. Breathe out all the way.
3. Hold your inhaler the way your doctor said (A, B, or C below).

Breathe in slowly

4. As you start breathing in **slowly** through your mouth, press down on the inhaler **one** time. (If you use a holding chamber, first press down on the inhaler. Within 5 seconds, begin to breathe in slowly.)
5. Keep breathing in **slowly**, as deeply as you can.

Hold your breath

6. Hold your breath as you count to 10 slowly, if you can.
7. For inhaled quick-relief medicine (beta$_2$-agonists), wait about 1 minute between puffs. There is no need to wait between puffs for other medicines.

A. Hold inhaler 1 to 2 inches in front of your mouth (about the width of two fingers).

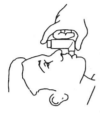

B. Use a spacer/holding chamber. These come in many shapes and can be useful to any patient.

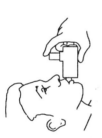

C. Put the inhaler in your mouth. Do not use for steroids.

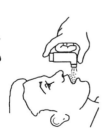

Clean Your Inhaler as Needed

Look at the hole where the medicine sprays out from your inhaler. If you see "powder" in or around the hole, clean the inhaler. Remove the metal canister from the L-shaped plastic mouthpiece. Rinse only the mouthpiece and cap in warm water. Let them dry overnight. In the morning, put the canister back inside. Put the cap on.

Know When To Replace Your Inhaler

For medicines you take each day (an example):
Say your new canister has 200 puffs (number of puffs is listed on canister) and you are told to take 8 puffs per day.

$$\begin{array}{r} 25 \text{ days} \\ 8 \text{ puffs per day} \overline{)\ 200 \text{ puffs in canister}} \end{array}$$

So this canister will last 25 days. If you started using this inhaler on May 1, replace it on or before May 25.

You can write the date on your canister.

For quick-relief medicine take as needed and count each puff.

Do not put your canister in water to see if it is empty. This does not work.

FIGURE 8.5. How to use metered-dose inhaler. (U.S. Department of Health and Human Services, National Institutes of Health. Practical guide for the diagnosis and management of asthma. NIH Publication No. 97-4053. Bethesda, MD: NIH.)

are more expensive than other delivery devices but may be essential for small children and during exacerbations. Inhaled steroids are not yet available for nebulizer use. Children approximately 3 years of age and older can be taught to use a spacer so that inhaled steroids may be prescribed.

PATIENT EDUCATION

Patient education is essential to good asthma management. The physician, parent, and patient should agree to goals for therapy, which usually include minimizing symptoms, a

☐ **Vacuum Cleaning**

- ☐ Try to get someone else to vacuum for you once or twice a week, if you can. Stay out of rooms while they are being vacuumed and for a short while afterward.
- ☐ If you vacuum, use a dust mask (from a hardware store), a double-layered or micro filter vacuum cleaner bag,* or a vacuum cleaner with a HEPA filter.*

☐ **Indoor Mold**

- ☐ Fix leaky faucets, pipes, or other sources of water.
- ☐ Clean moldy surfaces with a cleaner that has bleach in it.

☐ **Pollen and Outdoor Mold**

What to do during your allergy season (when pollen or mold spore counts are high):
- ☐ Try to keep your windows closed.
- ☐ Stay indoors with windows closed during the midday and afternoon, if you can. Pollen and some mold spore counts are highest at that time.
- ☐ Ask your doctor whether you need to take or increase anti-inflammatory medicine before your allergy season starts.

☐ **Smoke, Strong Odors, and Sprays**

- ☐ If possible, do not use a wood-burning stove, kerosene heater, or fireplace.
- ☐ Try to stay away from strong odors and sprays, such as perfume, talcum powder, hair spray, and paints.

☐ **Exercise, Sports, Work, or Play**

- ☐ You should be able to be active without symptoms. See your doctor if you have asthma symptoms when you are active—like when you exercise, do sports, play, or work hard.
- ☐ Ask your doctor about taking medicine before you exercise to prevent symptoms.
- ☐ Warm up for about 6 to 10 minutes before you exercise.
- ☐ Try not to work or play hard outside when the air pollution or pollen levels (if you are allergic to the pollen) are high.

☐ **Other Things That Can Make Asthma Worse**

- ☐ **Flu:** Get a flu shot.
- ☐ **Sulfites in foods:** Do not drink beer or wine or eat shrimp, dried fruit, or processed potatoes if they cause asthma symptoms.
- ☐ **Cold air:** Cover your nose and mouth with a scarf on cold or windy days.
- ☐ **Other medicines:** Tell your doctor about all the medicines you may take. Include cold medicines, aspirin, and even eye drops.

---

*To find out where to get products mentioned in this guide, call:

Asthma and Allergy Foundation of America (800-727-8462)

Allergy and Asthma Network/Mothers of

Asthmatics, Inc. (800-878-4403)

American Academy of Allergy, Asthma, and Immunology (800-822-2762)

National Jewish Medical and Research Center

FIGURE 8.6.   How to control factors that make asthma work. (U.S. Department of Health and Human Services, National Institutes of Health. Practical guide for the diagnosis and management of asthma. NIH Publication No. 97-4053. Bethesda, MD: NIH.)

convenient medication regimen, and avoidance of side effects. When asthma is first diagnosed, frequent visits for education may increase asthma understanding. Use of an asthma action plan (Fig. 8.4) facilitates good understanding of medication use, particularly when the child is receiving multiple medications. Medications may be particularly confusing for parents when generic preparations are used, as the appearance of the medication may change from month to month, and dosing instructions are usually printed on a box that is discarded when the inhaler is opened. Figure 8.6 discusses avoidance of factors that may exacerbate asthma. Compliance with allergen and irritant avoidance may be quite difficult, but this often results in marked improvement in control.

HOW TO CONTROL THINGS THAT MAKE YOUR ASTHMA WORSE

You can help prevent asthma attacks by staying away from things that make your asthma worse. This guide suggests many ways to help you do this.

You need to find out what makes your asthma worse. Some things that make asthma worse for some people are not a problem for others. You do not need to do all of the things listed in this guide.

Look at the things listed in dark print below. Put a check next to the ones that you know make your asthma worse. Ask your doctor to help you find out what else makes your asthma worse. Then, decide with your doctor what steps you will take. Start with the things in your <u>bedroom</u> that bother your asthma. Try something simple first.

☐   Tobacco Smoke

- ☐ If you smoke, ask your doctor for ways to help you quit. Ask family members to quit smoking, too.
- ☐ Do not allow smoking in your home or around you.
- ☐ Be sure no one smokes at a child's day care center.

☐   Dust Mites

Many people with asthma are allergic to dust mites. Dust mites are like tiny "bugs" you cannot see that live in cloth or carpet.

Things that will help the most:
- ☐ Encase your mattress in a special dust-proof cover.*
- ☐ Encase your pillow in a special dust-proof cover* or wash the pillow each week in hot water. Water must be hotter than 130^0F to kill the mites.
- ☐ Wash the sheets and blankets on your bed each week in hot water.

Other things that can help:
- ☐ Reduce indoor humidity to less than 50 percent. Dehumidifiers or central air conditioners can do this.
- ☐ Try not to sleep or lie on cloth-covered cushions or furniture.
- ☐ Remove carpets from your bedroom and those laid on concrete, if you can.
- ☐ Keep stuffed toys out of the bed or wash the toys weekly in hot water.

☐   Animal Dander

Some people are allergic to the flakes of skin or dried saliva from animals with fur or feathers.

The best thing to do:
- ☐ Keep furred or feathered pets out of your home.

If you can't keep the pet outdoors, then:
- ☐ Keep the pet out of your bedroom and keep the bedroom door closed.
- ☐ Cover the air vents in your bedroom with heavy material to filter the air.*
- ☐ Remove carpets and furniture covered with cloth from your home. If that is not possible, keep the pet out of the rooms where these are.

☐   Cockroach

Many people with asthma are allergic to the dried droppings and remains of cockroaches.

- ☐ Keep all food out of your bedroom.
- ☐ Keep food and garbage in closed containers (never leave food out).
- ☐ Use poison baits, powders, gels, or paste (for example, boric acid). You can also use traps.
- ☐ If a spray is used to kill roaches, stay out of the room until the odor goes away.

FIGURE 8.6. continued.

FOLLOW-UP

Frequency of follow-up depends on disease severity and caregiver comfort with the child's regimen. Well-controlled asthmatics are usually seen every 3 to 6 months, and during acute exacerbations. At these follow-up visits the exact medication regimen is reviewed. Overuse of beta agonists is a sign of poor asthmatic control and is associated with increased mortality from asthma. Unexpectedly frequent refills of beta agonist medications may be a sign of noncompliance with antiinflammatory medications. Missed school days, emergency room visits, or hospitalizations are reviewed. As coping with a chronically ill child and complicated treatment regimens can be quite stressful, family stress should be monitored. Medication side effects, especially behavioral, should be assessed. When the symptoms are well controlled, as evidenced by symptoms and peak flow readings consistently greater than 80% of predicted (green zone), the medications can be gradually stepped down. Annual influenza vaccination is recommended.

REFERRAL

Specialist referral depends on the experience and comfort of the physician with asthma, availability of specialty resources, comorbid conditions, and severity of the child's disease. Allergen immunotherapy may be a useful adjunct to therapy if an unavoidable allergen is identified. Counseling or other psychosocial intervention may be needed by some patients or families. If the child is very young or is not responding as expected to treatment, referral may be warranted.

REFERENCES

Abramson M, Puy R, Weiner J. Is allergen immunotherapy effective in asthma? A meta-analysis of randomised controlled trials. *Am J Respir Crit Care Med* 1995;151:969.

Calpin C, Macarthur C, Stephens D, Feldman W, Parkin PC. Effectiveness of prophylactic inhaled steroids in childhood asthma. *J Allergy Clin Immunol* 1997;100:452.

Kemper KJ. Chronic asthma: an update. *Pediatr Rev* 1996;17:111.

National Asthma Education and Prevention Program, National Heart, Lung and Blood Institute. Expert Panel Report 2. Clinical practice guidelines for the diagnosis and management of asthma. Bethesda, NIH Pub No. 97-4051, April 1997.

National Asthma Education and Prevention Program, National Heart, Lung and Blood Institute. Expert Panel Report 2. Practical guide for the diagnosis and management of asthma. Bethesda, NIH Pub No. 97-4053, October 1997.

Rabinovitch N, Gelfand EW. New approaches to the treatment of childhood asthma. *Curr Opin Pediatr* 1998;10:243.

Patient Education/Resources

American Lung Association. 800-LUNGUSA. www.lungusa.org. Patient education, camp directory.

Allergy and Asthma Network: Mothers of Asthmatics, Inc. 800-878-4403. www.aanma.org. Patient education, product directory.

Plaut TF. *Children with asthma: a manual for parents,* 2nd ed. Amherst, MA: Pedipress, 1998.

Type 1 Diabetes Mellitus

Family physicians frequently care for children with type 1 diabetes mellitus, formerly called insulin-dependent diabetes mellitus. Although pediatric endocrinologists may argue that these children should be referred to specialists, they may be cared for by the primary care physician, either because of patient or parental preference or because of the difficulties of frequent travel for specialty care. With the recent Diabetes Control and Complications Trial (DCCT) reporting a reduction in retinopathy, nephropathy, and neuropathy with tighter diabetic control, physicians who care for children with type 1 diabetes must strive to improve glucose levels while avoiding or treating the accompanying hypoglycemia.

Usually, the diagnosis of type I diabetes is straightforward. These children present with increased thirst, increased appetite, fatigue, and weight loss, urinary frequency or incontinence, or lethargy. Once the diagnosis is made, many children and adolescents are admitted to the hospital for initial education and management. Whether managed on an in patient or out patient basis, these patients and families go through the emotional stress of a lifelong illness, mourning the loss of a normal child, and fear of complications, all while trying to learn about insulin administration, glucose monitoring, and dietary management. During this stressful time, the physician needs to have patience and reemphasize important educational points. If management is especially difficult, it may indicate preexisting dysfunctional tendencies in the family that have been worsened by caring for the diabetic child.

HISTORY

Symptoms should be ascertained at follow-up visits. Is the patient having hypoglycemia or urinary frequency? Who is preparing the insulin injections? Are there concerns? How often is the glucose checked? What are the readings? Does the family have a glucagon emergency kit and urinary ketone strips, and have they familiarized themselves with their use? Are there dietary concerns? Any concerns regarding school? What is the child's usual level of exercise? How are the diet and insulin managed around exercise? Has the child seen a specialist (endocrinologist, ophthalmologist, dietitian, etc.)? How are the child and family coping emotionally with the illness? Particular attention is paid to visual, gastrointestinal, and urinary disturbances.

PHYSICAL EXAMINATION

The growth evaluation is one of the most important aspects of the physical examination. Excessive weight gain may be due to too much insulin, whereas insufficient insulin may lead to growth and developmental delay. Other aspects of the routine examination include the following:

Blood pressure (early marker of diabetic nephropathy)

Eye examination

Oral examination

Thyroid palpation

Cardiac examination

Abdominal examination

Palpation of peripheral pulses

Neurologic examination

Skin examination (especially glucose test sites)

Hand/finger examination

Foot examination

Beginning at least within 5 years of diagnosis, the child should have annual ophthalmologic evaluations, as early treatment of diabetic retinopathy reduces the risk of blindness. Sexual development may be delayed by poor diabetic control.

LABORATORY EVALUATION

At diagnosis, baseline creatinine, glycosylated hemoglobin (HbA1c), urinalysis, and thyroid stimulating hormone (TSH) are obtained. In children more than 2 years of age, a lipid profile is obtained at baseline and repeated once glycemic control is obtained. If the total cholesterol is less than 180 and LDL is less than 120, it is repeated every 5 years.

HbA1c reflects glycemic control over the preceding 3 months. It is usually measured every 3 months. Microalbumin is an early indicator of potential diabetic complications and is measured annually after puberty and 5 years of disease. Creatinine, TSH, and urinalysis should be rechecked periodically.

NUTRITIONAL MANAGEMENT

Dietary management is essential to good glycemic control. Yet achieving adequate understanding and compliance can be difficult. Day-to-day consistency in meal and snack times and caloric intake facilitates management. Daily caloric requirements vary widely, and may be best judged by the child's appetite in conjunction with close follow-up of growth. As an estimate, children require 1,000 calories for the first year of age and 100 calories per additional year for girls and 125 calories per year of age for boys. Depending on activity level, up to an additional 20% of the estimated calories may be needed. The standard diabetic diet contains 55% to 60% carbohydrate, 20% protein, and less than 30% fat, with less stringent fat restriction in the child under 2 years of age. If the child is on a regimen of two injections per day of NPH and Regular insulin, three meals and an evening snack are needed to avoid hypoglycemia from the peak effects of the insulin. In children on more intensive insulin regimens, snacks may not be needed. Individualized meal plans that take food preferences and individual schedules into account are developed with the help of a dietitian.

INSULIN THERAPY

Most children start with twice-daily insulin injections, one before breakfast, the other before dinner. This dose is usually initially divided two-thirds is given in the morning (2/3 NPH and 1/3 R) and one-third is given in the evening (split 1/2 NPH and 1/2 R). Soon after diagnosis many patients enter a "honeymoon period" in which exogenous insulin requirements are low, below 0.5 U/kg/day. The end of the honeymoon period is signaled by increasing insulin requirements and declining C-peptide levels. Following initiation of insulin, the dose is titrated upward, with most preadolescents requiring 0.75 to 1.0 U/kg/day and adolescents needing 1.0 to 1.2 U/kg/day. Table 8.7 lists commonly used insulins.

Insulin doses are adjusted based on blood glucose measurements and the duration and peak action of the insulin. At first this is done solely by the physician, but later

T ABLE 8.7. Insulins

Type	Onset (hours)	Peak (hours)	Duration of Action (hours)
Lispro (Humalog)	<0.25	1	3.5–4.5
Humulin Regular	0.5	2–4	6–80
Humulin NPH	1–2	6–12	18–24
Humulin Ultralente	4–6	8–20	24–48

the child and family learn to adjust the dose themselves. If the blood glucose is elevated in the morning, a 2 A.M. glucose should be measured to rule out hypoglycemia with overcompensation as the cause of the hyperglycemia.

INTENSIVE THERAPY

With the DCCT showing better outcomes with stricter control, intensive therapy has become more important. Some patients with regular eating habits and routines can achieve the goals of intensive treatment with the standard regimen; others cannot, because of variable exercise, diet, or routine. In these cases other insulin regimens (one-fifth of the total daily insulin dose given in the morning and afternoon) can be used to provide a basal amount of insulin with boluses of R or Humalog given before meals (one-fifth of the total daily dose each). These doses can be varied for glucose level and amount to be ingested. This regimen gives greater flexibility and often eliminates the need for an evening snack, but it requires frequent monitoring and multiple injections.

Insulin pumps also can accomplish intensive management. These also give a continuous basal insulin dose with as-needed boluses. They require a compliant patient who is willing and able to learn to use the device.

All intensive therapy increases the likelihood of hypoglycemic attacks.

MANAGEMENT GOALS

At first pass it would seem desirable to have all patients under intensive control with normal or nearly normal (HgbA1c). For young children, tight control is not usually possible, because of irregular diets and the difficulty in recognizing and treating hypoglycemia. For older children, the patient, family, and physician should develop realistic expectations, balancing the reduction in diabetic complications with the risk of hypoglycemia and frequency of monitoring and injections. Unrealistic goals may lead to inconsistent follow-up. With a therapeutic partnership, diabetes management can be maximized in the context of the individual family.

HYPOGLYCEMIA

Hypoglycemia results from either too much insulin, too much exercise, or ingestion of too few calories. Symptoms include confusion, irritability, severe hunger, lethargy, or in severe cases, loss of consciousness. Most children under 6 or 7 years of age have "hypoglycemic unawareness" in that they do not recognize the symptoms of hypoglycemia and must rely on caregivers for this recognition. If symptoms are present, the blood glucose should be measured. If it is less than 70 mg/dL, the child should be given 15 g of carbohydrate (e.g., five Life Savers, 2 tablespoons of raisins, 1/2 cup of regular soda). (Cake frosting may be easily carried away from home.) The glucose is

T ABLE 8.8. Sick-day management

Do not stop insulin
Increase fluids (3–6 ounces every half hour for young children and 6–8 ounces for older ones)
Measure blood glucose every 2–4 hours
Measure urinary ketones every 2–4 hours or with every void
If ketones are present, give supplemental short-acting insulin (10% of usual total daily dose) and repeat ketone
    measurement every 2–4 hours
If blood glucose is less than 150–200 mg/dL, use carbohydrate-containing fluids following the insulin bolus
If solids cannot be ingested, carbohydrate needs may be met with beverages such as juice or soda
Contact the physician if fluids are not tolerated, ketones persist following two insulin boluses, or there is
    worsening hyperglycemia, hypoglycemia, or ketosis

Adapted from Haire-Joshu D. Management of diabetes mellitus: perspectives of care across the lifespan, 2nd ed.
St.Louis, MO: Mosby, 1996.

repeated in 15 minutes, and if the sugar is still less than 70, the carbohydrate is
repeated. Special snacks such as cake or candy should not be used routinely for hypoglycemia, as they may encourage the child to desire hypoglycemia. Severe reactions
in which the child cannot ingest the carbohydrate or is unconscious are treated with
glucagon 1.0 mg (0.5 mg if the child weighs less than 20 kg) intramuscularly. This can
be repeated after 15 minutes if the child does not improve. Oral carbohydrates are
given once the child is able to take them. Following the event, the potential causes
are reviewed to avoid repeated hypoglycemia. Parents and caregivers should be
instructed on glucagon use with initial diabetic teaching.

SICK-DAY MANAGEMENT

Management of the ill child with type 1 diabetes can be especially challenging. Many
diabetics' natural tendency is to stop their insulin when they are ill, especially when
they are not eating normally, yet they may well have an increased need for insulin.
Sick-day management begins before the child is ill with education of the child and
caregivers. The rationale for continuing insulin is explained in detail. Table 8.8 outlines sick-day management.

T ABLE 8.9. Strategies for safe exercise

Blood glucose should be measured before exercise.
During prolonged exercise, glucose should be measured and if decreased, carbohydrates taken.
Hypoglycemia may occur up to 30 hours after strenuous or unaccustomed exercise, so glucose should be
    measured frequently.
Exercise is best tolerated 1–2 hours after a meal.
Exercise at the time of peak effect of the insulin dose is more likely to induce hypoglycemia.
Insulin should be injected into a nonexercising location (e.g., abdomen) if exercise will begin within 40 minutes
    after the injection.
Increase fluids (plain water if <60-minute event, sports drinks or half-strength fruit juice for longer ones).

Reprinted with permission from Haire-Joshu D. Management of diabetes mellitus: perspectives of care across the
lifespan, 2nd ed. St.Louis, MO: Mosby, 1996.

EXERCISE

Exercise can improve the health and well-being of diabetic children, yet strenuous activity requires increased attention to glycemic control to avoid hypoglycemia. Table 8.9 outlines strategies for successful exercise.

In young children exercise is often unpredictable, and so frequent monitoring after exercise is essential. Over time the athlete and caregivers generally become adept at predicting the individual's glycemic response to exercise and adjust insulin and diet accordingly.

DEVELOPMENTAL ISSUES

The young child's diabetes is generally managed by the caregiver. As the child matures, responsibility for diabetic management is gradually shifted to the patient. Teaching should be continuously repeated so that the child can assimilate it in greater depth as he or she matures.

Adolescents are notoriously difficult to manage. Information needs to be given in an informal and interactive way. Diabetic girls are particularly prone to eating disorders. Insulin requirements are generally increased, usually to 1.2 U/kg/day. Participation in summer camps may help the diabetic adolescent feel less "different" from peers. Patients may be concerned about sexual dysfunction yet afraid to ask. The increased risks associated with smoking for diabetics should be reemphasized. Many teens skip blood glucose monitoring and may fabricate results. The physician should seek to strengthen the relationship with the patient in the hopes of obtaining honest if not desirable information.

REFERRAL

The choice to refer a diabetic child depends on the individual physician's comfort with diabetic care as well as the availability and accessibility of these services. With the DCCT showing reduction in diabetic complications with intensive management, patients who desire this care should have it available to them, either with their family physician or with a specialist. Very young children are most difficult to manage and usually benefit from specialist referral.

REFERENCES

American Diabetes Association. Standards of Medical Care for Patients with Diabetes Mellitus. Clinical practice recommendations 1999.

Haire-Joshu, D. *Management of diabetes mellitus: perspectives of care across the lifespan,* 2nd ed. St Louis, MO: Mosby, 1996.

Jacobson AM. The psychological care of patients with insulin dependent diabetes mellitus. *N Engl J Med* 1996;334:1249.

Plotnick L. Insulin-dependent diabetes mellitus. *Pediatr Rev* 1994;15:137.

Tamborlane WV, Ahern J. Implications and result of the Diabetes Control and Complications Trial. *Pediatr Clin North Am* 1997;44:285.

Patient Education/Resources

American Diabetes Association. 800-DIABETES. www.diabetes.org. Provider and patient education materials. Summer camp clearinghouse.
International Juvenile Diabetes Foundation. 800-JDF-CURE.

Seminario L, Betschart J. *Raising a child with diabetes.* Alexandria, VA: American Diabetes Association, 1995.

Mental Retardation

Developmental delay may be anticipated through prenatal testing or diagnosed in the newborn period. Some children fail to meet developmental milestones and are diagnosed later in childhood. In all cases a thorough search for an identifiable etiology is indicated. The search for an identifiable cause should be reopened as new tests become available or if the child deteriorates. Family physicians can be the ideal source of support to the mentally retarded child and family.

HISTORY OF THE PRESENT ILLNESS

In many cases the history may be limited by the child's difficulty communicating. Many parents are especially attentive and may be very good historians; others may be unable to provide details. For children in residential care, only limited histories may be available. In general, the history is similar to other well-child visits, although the questions should be based on developmental rather than on chronologic age. Particular attention should be paid to the nutritional history as well as to bowel and bladder concerns. Physical and sexual abuse is more prevalent in this population and may be elicited by a sensitive history.

PAST MEDICAL HISTORY

In many cases the developmentally delayed child will have multiple concurrent medical and psychologic conditions. The family physician should receive updates on these conditions and help to coordinate specialty care.

SOCIAL HISTORY

Families may be severely stressed coping with a mentally retarded child, so coping mechanisms should be explored. Also, questions about school functioning are important. Clarification of guardianship may be needed, especially in older adolescents and children who do not live with their biologic parents.

PHYSICAL EXAMINATION

Because the history may be limited, the physical examination should be especially detailed. Growth should be plotted both on the standard growth chart and on a condition-specific growth chart when available. Vision and hearing screening should not be overlooked. Particular attention should be paid to the mouth, ear, cardiovascular, musculoskeletal, and dermatologic examination.

LABORATORY EVALUATION

Laboratory evaluation depends on the diagnosis. All children with mental retardation of undetermined etiology should have magnetic resonance imaging of the brain, metabolic screening and chromosomal analysis, generally including high-resolution chromosomal analysis and fragile X studies. This may have been previously omitted in older children and adults.

HEALTH MAINTENANCE

Hepatitis B is more common in mentally retarded individuals and so immunization is especially important. Hepatitis A vaccination should be especially considered in seronegative institutionalized patients. Pneumococcal and influenza vaccines should be considered if the child has repeated respiratory infections or lives in a setting with exposure to multiple disabled children. Pap smears may be especially difficult in the mentally retarded. If the adolescent has never been sexually active, screening is not generally needed, although a reliable sexual history may be difficult to obtain.

COMMON MEDICAL PROBLEMS

Psychiatric illness is very common in children with mental retardation. Unfortunately, distinguishing mental illness from the underlying condition can be especially difficult. Mental illness may present differently in the child with developmental disabilities. Alternatively, behavioral problems may be misdiagnosed as mental illness. Behaviors that may be expected at the child's developmental stage (e.g., imaginary friends) may be mistaken for a psychiatric disorder because of the child's chronologic age. Most mental health care providers receive little training in the nuances of diagnosis and treatment of mental illness in the mentally retarded. Consultants with this expertise should be sought out when possible, as many children respond well to appropriate behavioral and pharmacologic management.

Musculoskeletal

Many patients have musculoskeletal conditions, such as spasticity or hypotonia. Close cooperation with occupational therapists, physical therapists, and orthopedists may be needed to achieve maximum function. Atlantoaxial instability occurs in approximately 15% of children with Down syndrome. Symptoms include neck pain, abnormal gait, weakness or clumsiness of the arms, and abnormal reflexes. These symptoms may remain static for months or years and occasionally progress. Although clear evidence of benefit is lacking, lateral plain radiographs have long been recommended to screen for asymptomatic atlantoaxial instability in children with Down syndrome. Children with asymptomatic atlantoaxial instabililty are thought to be at increased risk of spinal cord injury during athletics and so their participation is restricted. At present this screening is required for participation in Special Olympics.

Genitourinary

Contraception may be difficult and controversial. The patient and guardian may need to give consent. States may have regulations concerning contraception or sterilization of the mentally retarded. These are usually available from the Office for Developmental Disabilities.

Gastrointestinal

Children with developmental delay are at risk for early feeding disorders. Breastfeeding may be especially important to decrease the risk of infection but often requires specialized support such as from a lactation consultant. Gastroesophageal reflux disease (GERD) is common and may present with respiratory symptoms. Obesity is common in older children and should be addressed proactively. Table 8.10 lists common medical problems associated with specific causes of mental retardation.

T ABLE 8.10. Common medical problems associated with specific causes of mental retardation

Down syndrome	Hearing loss, congenital heart disease, gastroesophageal reflux disease, constipation, hypothyroidism, dental disorders, seizures, atlantoaxial instability, hip dislocation, otitis media
Fragile X syndrome	Serous otitis media, mitral valve prolapse, strabismus, seizures, autism, language delay, hyperactivity, large head circumference, macroorchidism, flat feet
Fetal alcohol syndrome	Visual problems, serous otitis media, hearing loss, heart defects, urinary tract abnormalities, sensory hypersensitivity, growth retardation including microcephaly, hyperactivity, memory loss

ANTICIPATORY GUIDANCE

Parents of the developmentally disabled child need support from the physician. They may have feelings of guilt or inadequacy. Genetic testing may alleviate these feelings or may augment them by identifying the parent with a genetic defect. Genetic testing may provide valuable information regarding risk in future pregnancies. The child should be referred to early intervention programs as soon as possible after diagnosis. Mainstreaming has become increasingly common in schools, but these children may be socially isolated nevertheless. As children and parents age, arrangements for guardianship and financial support should be made.

REFERRAL

The need for referral is determined by the child's condition, local resources, and physician's comfort in managing the child. At diagnosis referral often facilitates identification of the underlying etiology or syndrome.

FOLLOW-UP

Follow-up is individualized. Older children are prone to being lost to follow-up and should be seen at least annually.

PATIENT EDUCATION/RESOURCES

American Association on Mental Retardation. www.aamr.org. 800-424-3688

National Down Syndrome Society. www.ndss.org. 800-221-4602.

National Fragile X Foundation. 800-688-8765. www.fragileX.org.

National Organization on Fetal Alcohol Syndrome. 800-66NOFOS. www.nofas.org.

Down syndrome. Handout available from AAFP online at www.familydoctor.org.

REFERENCES

Committee on Genetics. American Academy of Pediatrics. Health supervision for children with Down syndrome. *Pediatrics* 1994;93:855.

Committee on Genetics. American Academy of Pediatrics. Health supervision for children with fragile X syndrome. *Pediatrics* 1996;98:297.

Committee on Sports Medicine and Fitness. American Academy of Pediatrics. Atlantoaxial instability in Down syndrome: subject review. *Pediatrics* 1995;96:151.

Committee on Substance Abuse and Committee on Children with Disabilities. American Academy of Pediatrics. Fetal alcohol syndrome and fetal alcohol effects. *Pediatrics* 1993;91:1004.

Hagerman R. Fragile X syndrome. In: Parker S, Zuckerman B, eds. *Behavioral and developmental pediatrics.* Boston: Little, Brown, 1995:153.

Hurley AD. Psychiatric disorders in children and adolescents with mental retardation and developmental delay. *Curr Opin Pediatr* 1996;8:361.

Martin BA. Primary care of adults with mental retardation living in the community. *Am Fam Physician* 1997;56:485.

Morse BA, Weiner L. Fetal alcohol syndrome. In: Parker S, Zuckerman B, eds. *Behavioral and developmental pediatrics.* Boston: Little, Brown, 1995:149.

Saenz RB. Primary care of infants and young children with Down syndrome. *Am Fam Physician* 1999;59:381.

Human Immunodeficiency Virus

Although some may argue that care of the child exposed to the human immunodeficiency virus (HIV) or the child infected by it is best left to pediatric HIV specialists, family physicians may be called on to care for these children. As most children acquire HIV from their mothers, the families of these children are often coping with the parent's illness as well as the child's. These families may not have the financial resources or the transportation for specialty care, especially in rural areas. Many family physicians have experience treating HIV-infected adults, which acquaints them with the management of this disease. HIV care changes very frequently, and so care of these children requires frequent consultation with HIV specialists, either in person or via the phone. The new antiretrovirals require extremely high levels of compliance. Family physicians with our relationships with the families may be best able to coordinate this care.

NEONATES

Pregnant women should be offered HIV testing during pregnancy. If this testing is positive, the mother and child benefit from antiretroviral therapy of the mother. Studies using zidovudine (AZT, Retrovir) have shown dramatic reductions in the rate of infection of the neonate. Combination antiretroviral therapy is usually recommended and is likely to improve on this success. Even if the mother did not receive prenatal antiretroviral therapy, intrapartum zidovudine prophylaxis can decrease the perinatal transmission rate.

Eight to 12 hours after birth, zidovudine prophylaxis should be started at 2 mg/kg every 6 hours and continued for 6 weeks. (The dose is adjusted for premature infants and infants with hepatic and renal dysfunction.) As HIV has been found in breast milk, these children should not breastfeed, except in countries where safe artificial formula is not available.

With viral load testing, HIV infection can be detected in most infants by 1 month of age. The HIV DNA polymerase chain reaction (PCR) or viral load should be measured at 48 hours, 2 weeks, 1 to 2 months, and 3 to 6 months. If any test is positive, it should be repeated. If the test is confirmed as positive, the child is infected with the HIV virus. If two tests performed at greater than 1 month of age and one test performed beyond the age of 4 months are negative, HIV can be reasonably excluded. At age 18 months if the child has had negative viral loads, has a negative HIV IgG, and has no hypogammaglobulinemia and no signs of infection, HIV infection is definitively excluded (Guidelines for the Use of Antiretrovirals).

If the child tests positive, zidovudine therapy should be replaced with a combination antiretroviral regimen. The current preferred regimens include two nucleoside analog reverse transcriptase inhibitors (NRTIs) and a protease inhibitor. Because these regimens change frequently and have side effects, consultation with an HIV specialist is usually needed at this point. Because these children are recently infected, the regimens should be begun soon after diagnosis, as early treatment may improve efficacy. As with all combination antiretroviral regimens, perfect compliance is needed for maximum efficacy. Caregivers need to be fully instructed in the regimen, with frequent follow-up to ensure that the medications are being given correctly. In general, the regimen should be delayed if compliance cannot be assured. The new Guidelines for the Use of Antiretroviral Agents in Pediatric HIV Infection from the Centers for Disease Control give details of the preferred and alternative regimens as well as the dosing and side effects of the medications. These guidelines also give recommendations on when to change antiretroviral regimens.

Ideal nutrition is very important for HIV-infected children as it enhances their quality of life, their immune function, and the action of the antiretrovirals. As the $CD4^+$ count changes with the age of the child, the $CD4^+$ percentage more accurately reflects disease progression in children and is used to track immune function.

IMMUNIZATIONS

Varicella vaccine is not currently recommended in HIV-infected children. Measles-mumps-rubella (MMR) vaccine should be withheld in severely immunosuppressed HIV-infected children but may be given in infected children without severe immunosuppression. Inactivated polio vaccine (IPV) is recommended for HIV-infected children and their contacts. Other immunizations are given as in noninfected children. The schedule for immunizations is the same as that for noninfected individuals. Pneumococcal vaccine is recommended at 2 years of age, and annual influenza immunizations should begin at the age of 6 months. HIV-infected children exposed to measles or varicella virus generally require passive immunization with the appropriate immune globulin.

FOLLOW-UP

Children infected with HIV need serial laboratory evaluations. Usually the $CD4^+$ percentage and viral load are measured every 3 months. The complete blood count should be monitored frequently, especially in children receiving trimethoprim-sulfamethoxazole (Bactrim, Septra). Quantitative immunoglobulins can be measured to

T ABLE 8.11. Common complications of pediatric HIV infection

Poor weight gain and growth
Developmental delay
Neurologic conditions (seizures, mental retardation, cerebral palsy)
Pneumocystis carinii pneumonia
Lymphocytic interstitial pneumonitis
Candidal infection (diaper rash, thrush)
More frequent and severe common childhood bacterial infections

assess level of immunosuppression. Lower levels indicate greater immunosuppression. Other monitoring depends on the clinical condition and medications. Table 8.11 lists most common complications of HIV disease in children.

PNEUMOCYSTIS CARINII PNEUMONIA PROPHYLAXIS

Because most cases of *Pneumocystis carinii* pneumonia (PCP) in HIV-infected infants occur in the first year of life, PCP prophylaxis should be started at 4 to 6 weeks of age in all HIV-exposed infants. This may be discontinued at the age of 4 months if two viral load measurements have been negative. The usual regimen is trimethoprim-sulfamethoxazole: 5 mg/kg/day of trimethoprim and 25 mg/kg/day sulfamethoxazole divided into two daily doses and given for three consecutive days (e.g., Monday, Tuesday, Wednesday) each week.

In the HIV-infected infant, prophylaxis should be continued at least until the age of 1 year. Prophylaxis should be continued lifelong in a child with a history of PCP. In other children prophylaxis may be discontinued if the CD4+ percentage has always been above 15% and should be restarted if the CD4+ percentage drops below 15%.

OTHER OPPORTUNISTIC INFECTIONS

Tuberculosis testing with a PPD should be done annually beginning at the age of 1 year. This is considered positive if the induration is greater than 5 mm. If active tuberculosis is suspected, a negative PPD does not rule out infection. These children, as well as those exposed to patients with active tuberculosis, require individualized management. Prophylaxis against other opportunistic infections should be decided on a case-by-case basis. Typically, other prophylaxis is recommended following a documented opportunistic infection.

ANTICIPATORY GUIDANCE

Table 8.12 lists common anticipatory guidance for the HIV-infected child.

PSYCHOSOCIAL ISSUES

Families who have an HIV-infected child often are coping with multiple other stressors. Often one or more parent may be infected with or have died from HIV. If the caregiver is infected, custody arrangements may need to be discussed and arranged for the children. In general, the school-aged child should be informed of his or her condition. The physician should discuss the risks and benefits of disclosing the child's condition with school and day care personnel.

T ABLE 8.12. Anticipatory guidance

Avoid eating raw or uncooked food
Don't drink or swim in lake, pond, or river water
Avoid contact with young farm animals
Don't change cat litter boxes
Use good hand washing
Don't share tooth brushes

ADOLESCENT ISSUES

Most adolescents infected with HIV contracted the disease through sexual contact or drug abuse and are generally managed like adults with early HIV infection. The small though increasing number who contracted the disease early and survive to adolescence may follow their own unique clinical course and should be managed in consultation with HIV specialists familiar with their care. Adolescents commonly see themselves as invincible and so may deny their condition and be noncompliant with treatment. As antiretrovirals require extreme compliance, they should not be initiated until the provider is confident the adolescent understands and will comply. Close follow-up is essential. Precautions to prevent infection of others need to be emphasized.

PROGNOSIS

Before the availability of effective treatment, children infected perinatally with HIV had a median survival of 8 or 9 years. Twenty percent of these perinatally infected children had rapid disease progression, including severe immune suppression in the first 2 years of life. Intermediate progression, or severe immune suppression occurring by the age of 7 or 8 years, was seen in 60%. Another 20% were slow progressors, where few symptoms were seen by the age of 9 years. New studies are beginning to show increased AIDS-free survival in children treated with combination antiretrovirals, although documention of the full effect of current medication regimens will require years of study.

REFERENCES

American Academy of Pediatrics. Committee on Pediatric AIDS. Evaluation and medical treatment of the HIV exposed infant. *Pediatrics* 1997;99:909.

Centers for Disease Control. Guidelines for the use of antiretroviral agents in pediatric HIV infection. *MMWR* 1998;47(RR-4):1. Updated March 1999.

Centers for Disease Control. 1995 Revised guidelines for prophylaxis against *Pneumocystis carinii* pneumonia for children infected with or perinatally exposed to human immunodeficiency virus. *MMWR* 1995;44(RR-4):1.

Centers for Disease Control. 1997 USPHS/IDSA guidelines for the prevention of opportunistic infections in persons infected with human immunodeficiency virus. *MMWR* 1997;46(RR-4):1.

Luzuriaga K, Sullivan JL. Prevention and treatment of pediatric HIV infection. *JAMA* 1998;280:17.

Rogers MF, ed. HIV/AIDS in infants, children and adolescents. *Pediatr Clinics of North America* 2000;47:1.

Patient Education/Resources

The San Francisco General Warmline. 800-933-3413. Clinical consultation for health care providers available weekdays.

Centers for Disease Control and Prevention. www.cdc.gov.

AIDS Treatment Information Service. 800-HIV-8440. www.hivatis.org. Management protocols, clinical trials.

AIDS Clinical Trials Information Service. 800-TRIALS-A. www.actis.org.

National AIDS Hotline, open 24 hours, 7 days a week. 800-342-AIDS.

National Pediatric and Family HIV Resource Center (University of Medicine and Dentistry of New Jersey). www.pedhivaids.org.

National Pediatric HIV Resource Center. 800-362-0071.

Sande MA, Gilbert DN, Moellering RC. The Sanford Guide to HIV/AIDS Therapy. Published annually, inexpensive, similar format to Sanford Guide to Antimicrobial Therapy. Order from:

Antimicrobial Therapy Inc.
Box 70
Hyde Park, VT 05655
802-888-2855

Premature Infant

Premature infants are defined as those born before 37 weeks' gestational age. Low-birth-weight infants weigh less than 2,500 g, whereas very-low-birth-weight infants weigh less than 1,500 g. Survival is improving, especially for the most premature infants, and so family physicians may need to care for tinier children. Before discharge from the Neonatal Intensive Care Unit (NICU) the infant must meet criteria that ensure that he or she can be cared for safely at home (Table 8.13).

HISTORY

The NICU discharge summary should be available to the physician, ideally before the first office visit. This summary should include the patient's treatment while in the NICU, current medications, and immunization history. Anticipated follow-up needs may be outlined. The first office visit should occur a few days after discharge. During the office visit the physician should ask the parents about the NICU course and clarify any questions. Because parents are highly stressed while their child is in the NICU, they may have been unable to understand the medical information they received. Parents should describe medications; treatments; type, amount, and frequency of feedings; monitor use; and travel arrangements. They should also outline in-home services and planned specialty follow-up. Sleep patterns should be described. Premature infants sleep more hours per day than full-term ones, but they tend to sleep fewer consecutive hours. This may add to the parental stress. Parents of premature infants report high stress, especially in the first months after bringing the child home. Depression, anxiety, and obsessive-compulsive behaviors are much more common

T ABLE 8.13. Common criteria for NICU discharge

Ability to maintain body temperature fully clothed in an open crib (usually at 34 weeks or 2,000 g)
Feeds adequately by mouth to gain 20–30 g/day
Stable cardiorespiratory function
No recent major changes in medications or oxygen delivery
Parents can provide for the infant's physical needs, including financially
Parents can identify problems that may arise after discharge
Defined plan for follow-up medical care and parenting support

than in parents of term infants. By the time the child is 3 years old, though, these symptoms are comparable to those of parents of term infants (Singer).

PHYSICAL EXAMINATION

The child's length, weight, and head circumference should be recorded at each visit. Special growth charts are available to plot these children's growth, as it varies from that of the term infant. These charts are usually available from the intensive care nursery, textbooks on premature infants, or Ross Pediatrics. With catch-up growth, the head grows first, followed by the weight and then the length. As these children are prone to hypertension, the blood pressure should be measured at least twice in the first year. This may be done by Doppler or palpation. (The Trachtenbarg reference lists normal values.) Head flattening usually resolves spontaneously but may be reduced by slight alterations in head position while supine. Nevertheless, the child should sleep supine to reduce the risk of sudden infant death syndrome (SIDS). The mouth should be inspected for dental anomalies or a high palatal vault, which are complications of oral intubation. Respiratory rate and pattern as well as the presence of abnormal lung sounds such as wheezing should be carefully assessed. The detailed neurologic examination includes assessment of postural reflexes, muscle tone, cranial nerves, sensory responses, and behavior. Early neurologic referral is indicated if any abnormalities are suspected. Undescended testes and inguinal hernias are more common than in term infants. The remainder of the examination is similar to that of the term infant.

DEVELOPMENT

Developmental assessment, using a screening tool such as the Denver Developmental Screen, is critical for these children. During the first 2 years, the child is plotted using the age past the due date. If abnormalities are detected, a formal development assessment, possibly by a developmental pediatrician, should be undertaken. Referral to early intervention programs may be helpful.

NUTRITION

Typical graduates of the NICU require 100 kcal/kg/day (unfortified breast milk and standard formula contain 20 kcal/ounce). Infants fed formula containing greater than 24 kcal/ounce are prone to hyperosmolarity. They should be watched carefully for signs of dehydration, especially if they develop vomiting or diarrhea. Electrolyte levels may need to be monitored. Generally, the infant can be changed to regular formula or unfortified breast milk at the due date, although special dietary intervention may be needed in the sicker infants. As breastfeeding has been shown to protect against infection and to improve development, mothers should be encouraged to continue nursing. Infants generally nurse every 2 or 3 hours and should not go more than 4 hours between feedings. The child should have six to eight wet diapers per day. Milk supply can be enhanced by pumping after feedings. A supplemental nurser, which delivers fluids through a tube adjacent to the nipple, can enhance caloric intake. Lactation consultants can be invaluable. Solid foods should be introduced 4 to 6 months after the due date. Formula should be continued until at least 12 months of age, longer for small-for-gestational-age and sick infants with catch-up growth. Breast milk should be continued as long as desired by the mother and child. Because the premature infant has lower iron stores than the term infant, iron supplementation is needed. The usual dose is 2 to 4 mg/kg beginning 2 weeks after birth and continuing to 1 year of age. Iron suspensions (i.e., Fer-in-Sol) contain 15 mg/0.6 mL. Additional iron is generally not needed in infants consuming iron-fortified formula. Vitamin D supplementation using a standard infant vitamin containing 400 IU/day is recommended for breastfeeding infants and those not yet consuming 32 ounces of formula per day. Supplementation may also be needed with some specialized formulas, which do not contain adequate vitamins.

FOLLOW-UP

At first, children are seen weekly. Once adequate growth and adaptation to home are ensured, these visits can become less frequent. The frequency of subsequent visits will depend on the child's medical problems as well as the frequency of specialty follow-up.

ANTICIPATORY GUIDANCE

Travel
Before discharge from the NICU the infant should be tested for apnea, bradycardia, or oxygen desaturation while in the car seat. If these complications are observed, travel either prone or supine in a specialized car safety device is recommended. Infants on apnea monitors should travel with them. Rolled towels may be needed either around the child's head or beneath the foot of the seat to keep the child positioned correctly.

Parental Stress
The birth of a premature child can be extremely stressful for parents, siblings, and extended families. Mothers have been shown to be more prone to depression, anxiety, and obsessive-compulsive disorders. The physician should be alert for early symptoms and begin treatment or arrange referral.

Health Maintenance
Immunizations are given based on the child's chronologic age, not the gestational age, and are given at the usual dose. The only exception is the hepatitis B vaccine, which is delayed until the child reaches 2,000 g (Losonsky). Respiratory syncytial virus immune globulin palivizumab [synagis] has been shown to prevent severe respiratory syncytial virus (RSV) infection. It should be considered in infants with bronchopulmonary dysplasia who are currently receiving oxygen therapy or have received it in the past 6 months and in infants born before 32 weeks. (See the full AAP statement for exact indications and dosing.) Hearing screening using a brainstem auditory response is generally completed before discharge from the NICU. If parents report concerns about hearing or with language delay, hearing should be reassessed.

COMMON MEDICAL PROBLEMS

Developmental disability is the most feared complication of prematurity. It occurs in 10% to 20% of preterm infants with a weight of less than 1,500 g, usually in the setting of intraventricular hemorrhage, especially grade 3 or 4, or periventricular leukomalacia. As hypoxic injury tends to be diffuse, evidence of one developmental abnormality should prompt a search for others, usually by a multidisciplinary team. In preterm infants without intraventricular hemorrhage, periventricular leukomalacia, or ventricular dilation, the risk of developmental delay is not greater than that for term infants. Developmental delay is uncommon in children who are meeting developmental milestones at the due date, although vigilance for learning disabilities, which may present later, is advised.

Apnea

Significant apnea is defined as lasting greater than 15 seconds, whereas periodic breathing is apnea that lasts from 5 to 15 seconds. Apnea monitoring is of unproven benefit in preventing sudden infant death syndrome (SIDS) but is commonly instituted in premature infants. Indications for monitoring include the following:

Less than 34 weeks' gestation at birth

Significant apnea not associated with a reversible illness

A sibling with SIDS

Bronchopulmonary dysplasia

Intraventricular hemorrhage

Parents of children with apnea monitors should be instructed in infant cardiopulmonary resuscitation (CPR). Newer monitors may record the heart rate during the apnea. A deceleration in heart rate followed by acceleration can distinguish a true apnea from monitor malfunction. Theophylline (3 to 5 mg/kg every 8 hours to maintain serum level 8 to 12 μg/mL) may improve the apnea. Usually, the monitor is discontinued when the child has no apnea associated with cyanosis or bradycardia for 2 months and no apnea requiring vigorous stimulation for 3 months. Other common medical problems for premature infants are discussed in Table 8.14.

REFERENCES

American Academy of Pediatrics, Committee on Infectious Diseases and Committee on the Fetus and the Newborn. Respiratory syncytial virus immune globulin intravenous indications for use. *Pediatrics* 1997;99:645.

American Academy of Pediatrics, Committee on the Fetus and the Newborn. Hospital discharge of the high-risk neonate: proposed guidelines. *Pediatrics* 1998;102:411.

American Academy of Pediatrics, Committee on Injury and Poison Prevention and Committee on the Fetus and the Newborn. Safe transportation of premature and low birth weight infants. *Pediatrics* 1996;97:758.

Losonsky GA, et al. Hepatitis B immunization of premature infants: a reassessment of current recommendations for delayed immunization. *Pediatrics* 1999;103:E14.

Singer LT, et al. Maternal psychological distress and parenting stress after the birth of a very low birth weight infant. *JAMA* 1999;281:799.

Spitzer AR. Intensive care of the fetus and newborn. St Louis, MO: Mosby, 1996.

Trachtenbarg DE, Goleman TB. Care of the premature infant: part I. Monitoring growth and development. *Am Fam Physician* 1998;57:2123.

Trachtenbarg DE, Goleman TB. Care of the premature infant: part II. Common medical and surgical problems. *Am Fam Physician* 1998;57:2383.

Resources

Ross Pediatrics. 800-227-5767. Supplier of premature infant growth charts.

TABLE 8.14. Premature infant

Medical Problem	Follow-up/Treatment	Comments
Undescended testes	Surgical referral at age 1 year	More common in premature infants
Inguinal hernia	Immediate surgical referral	High risk of incarceration
Intraventricular hemorrhage	Watch head growth closely. May need ultrasound to rule out hydrocephalus	Developmental delay common, especially in grade 3 or 4 hemorrhage
Gastroesophageal reflux disease	Smaller, more frequent feedings; H₂ blockers (Zantac 2–5 mg/kg twice a day)	May present as regurgitation, apnea, wheezing, worsened chronic lung disease (bronchopulmonary dysplasia)
Retinopathy of prematurity	High-risk infants are screened in the NICU, with follow-up schedule determined by initial findings	Cryotherapy and laser treatment reduce the risk of retinal detachment and blindness
Chronic lung disease (formerly designated bronchopulmonary dysplasia)	Usually managed in conjunction with a neonatologist; treatment may include hypercaloric formula, fluid restriction, diuretics, bronchodilators	Much less common with surfactant use. Oxygen saturations >95% promotes better weight gain, development, and reduces the risk of pulmonary hypertension and respiratory illness. Many cases could be prevented by prenatal steroid therapy.
Seizures	Usually require anticonvulsant therapy	Patients should have a normal electroencephalogram and be seizure-free for 3 months before medication withdrawal is considered.

Used with permission from Trachtenbarg DE, Golemon TB. Office care of the premature infant, Part II: common medical and surgical problems. *Am Fam Physician* 1998;57:2383.

Obesity

CHIEF COMPLAINT

"My child is overweight."

HISTORY

The history begins with assessment of the child's growth, from either the growth chart or the parent's recollection. The parents or child should record when they noticed the weight problem. Previous attempts at weight reduction should be noted. A detailed dietary history should be taken that includes typical daily intake of meals and snacks. This may be facilitated by a few-day diary of intake. Periods of overeating should be explored. Frequency and type of exercise should be assessed. Signs of sleep apnea such as daytime somnolence and loud snoring should be elicited. Menstrual disorders are more common in obese adolescents.

PAST MEDICAL HISTORY

Hypothyroidism, Cushing's syndrome, pseudohypoparathyroidism, growth hormone deficiency, and syndromes such as Prader-Willi may lead to obesity. Medications, especially antipsychotics, may lead to weight gain.

FAMILY HISTORY

Obesity certainly runs in families. Twin studies show that this is due to genetic factors as well as behavioral ones. If applicable, parents' guilt about their own failed weight loss attempts or their "bad genes" should be addressed.

SOCIAL HISTORY

Obesity may lead to disrupted peer interactions. Overweight children are more prone to depression and low self-esteem. Many people, including physicians, inappropriately assume that obesity is the result of poor self-control.

PHYSICAL EXAMINATION

In general, a child who appears obese is in fact obese. In children weight alone is an inadequate gauge of obesity, as weight varies with height. Weight greater than 20% over ideal for height is often defined as obesity. Body mass index is calculated by dividing weight in kilograms by the square of the height in meters. Obesity is defined as a body mass index of greater than the 95th percentile for age. This value is 30 for late teens, lower for younger children. Abnormal appearance consistent with a genetic syndrome should be noted. Careful measurement of weight and height is essential, as short stature may indicate an underlying endocrine or genetic condition. Blood pressure may need to be measured with a large cuff. Skin conditions, such as tinea, intertrigo, and heat rash, are more common in very obese children. Orthopedic problems, especially joint problems in the lower extremities, are more frequent.

LABORATORY EVALUATION

No laboratory evaluation is generally needed in the evaluation of the obese child, unless the child has an abnormal appearance consistent with an endocrine or genetic syndrome, short stature, or decreased intelligence. Since hyperlipidemia augments cardiovascular risk, a lipid profile may be considered.

DIFFERENTIAL DIAGNOSIS

An underlying cause for obesity is found in only about 5% of children.

MANAGEMENT

The success rate for the management of childhood obesity is disappointing. Unfortunately, 80% of obese adolescents become obese adults, and these adults have higher morbidity and mortality than obese adults who were not obese in adolescence. Any successful treatment plan must include changes in activity as well as diet. In 20% of children weight reduction can be attained by decreasing soda, juice, and excess milk in the diet. High-fat and calorie-laden foods should be minimized and are best not kept in the home. Alternative snacks, such as sliced vegetables, should be readily available. Many patients confuse low-fat and low-calorie foods. To reduce weight, total calories as well as total fat must be reduced. Rigorous calorie counting may lead some patients to reduce intake. Others find this unacceptable. Not eating while watching television, taking smaller bites, chewing more, and leaving food on the plate at the end of the meal may help. If the child overeats when stressed, stress reduction measures should be explored.

Combining increased physical activity with decreased dietary intake is more effective than the dietary intervention alone. This is supported by recent evidence suggesting that decreased energy expenditure may play a larger role in weight gain in children than increased energy intake (Schonfeld). Emphasizing reduced inactivity rather than increased activity seems to be more effective at improving vigorous activity. Table 8.15 lists examples of methods to reduce inactivity.

Weight goals depend on the age of the child. In the mildly obese prepubertal child, weight maintenance may eliminate obesity as the child grows. A healthy weight is up to 20% above or below ideal height for weight. Adolescents may safely lose 1 or 2 pounds a week while trying to achieve this goal. Although, if this goal is very distant, setting a goal of a modest weight reduction of 10 pounds may be a better first step. Positive reinforcement is essential. Success rates improve if the whole family joins in the effort of weight reduction. Frequent small rewards are more effective than prolonged waits for larger ones. Achievable weekly goals for diet and activity should be

T ABLE 8.15. Methods to reduce inactivity

Reduce time spent watching television
Reduce time on the computer or on computer games
Use stairs instead of elevators
Play outside instead of inside

Adapted from Schonfeld-Warden N, Warden CH. Pediatric obesity: an overview of etiology and treatment. *Pediatr Clin North Am* 1997;44:339.

T ABLE 8.16. Preventing obesity: tips for parents

Respect your child's appetite: children do not need to finish every bottle or meal.
Avoid pre-prepared and sugared foods when possible.
Limit the amount of high-calorie foods kept in the home.
Provide a healthy diet, with 30% or fewer calories derived from fat.
Provide ample fiber in the child's diet.
Skim milk may safely replace whole milk at 2 years of age.
Do not provide food for comfort or as a reward.
Do not offer sweets in exchange for a finished meal.
Limit amount of television viewing.
Encourage active play.
Establish regular family activities such as walks, ball games, and other outdoor activities.

From Moran R. Evaluation and treatment of childhood obesity. *Am Fam Physician* 1999;59:861. Used with permission.

established. Small victories should be celebrated. Criticism and punishment are ineffective. Weight should be measured at most weekly, to emphasize behavioral change.

Many experts are emphasizing the role of obesity prevention since treatment has been so difficult. Family physicians can easily recognize high-risk families and recommend changes in diet and activity in these children. Table 8.16 lists methods for parents to prevent obesity.

FOLLOW-UP

Follow-up depends on the intensity of the intervention. If the child and family have embarked on a major behavioral change, weekly follow-up is essential. At follow-up visits activity logs can be reviewed. Children and parents should be liberally praised for any improvements. If the child is successful in reducing obesity, continued reinforcement at future visits, even those for acute problems, is helpful. Follow-up phone calls from office staff can be helpful.

REFERRAL

Referral to a dietitian may facilitate education of child and family regarding lower-calorie diets. Support groups may help with improving motivation. In very obese children and adolescents where other interventions have failed, referral to specialty centers for protein-sparing modified fasts may be considered. The Shapedown Pediatric Obesity Program is a structured weight-loss program for the 6- to 20-year age group and has offices throughout the country. The Weight-Control Information Network is a clearinghouse for weight reduction information for providers and patients.

REFERENCES

Barlow SE, Dietz WH. Obesity evaluation and treatment: expert committee recommendations. *Pediatrics* 1998;102:E29.

Hammer L. Obesity. In: Parker S, Zuckerman B, eds. *Behavioral and developmental pediatrics.* Boston: Little, Brown, 1995:223.

Moran R. Evaluation and treatment of childhood obesity. *Am Fam Physician* 1999; 59:861.

Schonfeld-Warden N, Warden CH. Pediatric obesity: an overview of etiology and treatment. *Pediatr Clin North Am* 1997;44:339.

Patient Education

Helping your child keep a healthy weight. Handout available from AAFP online at www.familydoctor.org.

Helping your child lose weight. Handout available from AAFP online at www.familydoctor.org.

Epstein LH, Squires S. The stoplight diet for children: an eight-week program for parents and children. Boston: Little, Brown, 1988.

Shapedown. 415-453-8886. www.shapedown.com.

Weight Control Information Network. 800-946-8098. www.niddk.nih.gov/health/nutrit/pubs/win.htm.

•••

CHAPTER 9

Psychiatric Conditions

Attention-Deficit Hyperactivity Disorder

CHIEF COMPLAINT

"My child is doing poorly in school." "The teacher wants my child evaluated for attention deficit."

HISTORY OF PRESENT ILLNESS

The history is the most critical element in the evaluation of a child for possible attention deficit/hyperactivity disorder (ADHD). Information is usually gathered from parents, counselors, teachers, other school officials (including the school psychologist), and others in contact with the child. Schools are federally mandated to evaluate children who are suspected of having ADHD or a learning disorder that impairs academic functioning, although the school may need reminding. All evaluations should be available for the physician at the time of the office visit. Table 9.1 is an ADHD symptom checklist. This information should be compiled from the multiple sources, often by an office nurse. The physician should also ask about any previous medication use, including why they were stopped and any side effects. Since enuresis and encopresis are common in children being evaluated for ADHD, this history should be specifically elicited.

PAST MEDICAL HISTORY

ADHD is more common in children with developmental disorders. The physician should ask about a history of fetal alcohol exposure, lead exposure, or head injury. Table 9.2 lists medical conditions that may mimic ADHD.

FAMILY HISTORY

A child is at greater risk for ADHD when there is a family history of ADHD in the siblings or parents. It is also important to elicit a family history of behavioral disorders, psychiatric disorders, tics, and learning disorders.

SOCIAL HISTORY

The social history is a particularly important aspect of the evaluation. The physician should be aware of the members of the household, particular stressors, especially substance abuse and domestic abuse; and remedial educational interventions already in place. Families are often negatively affected by the ADHD, and so the effect of the ADHD on other family members, especially siblings, should be sought out.

T ABLE 9.1. Symptom checklist

Child's Name: _____ Age: _____ Date: _____
Person(s) completing form: _____ Relationship: _____
Setting: _____ Time/Subject: _____

Check the box that best describes this child compared with other children of the same gender and age.	Never	Sometimes	Often	Very often
Scale A:				
1. Fails to pay close attention to details or makes careless mistakes in schoolwork, chores, or other tasks	N	S	O	VO
2. Has difficulty sustaining attention to tasks, chores, or activities	N	S	O	VO
3. Does not seem to listen when spoken to directly	N	S	O	VO
4. Does not follow through on instructions and fails to finish schoolwork, chores, or duties (not due to oppositional behavior or failure to understand directions)	N	S		VO
5. Has difficulty organizing tasks and activities	N	S	O	VO
6. Avoids, dislikes, or is reluctant to engage in tasks that require sustained mental effort (such as schoolwork)	N	S	O	VO
7. Loses things necessary for tasks or activities (eg, toys, school assignments, pencils, books, or tools)	N	S	O	VO
8. Is distracted by unimportant stimuli	N	S	O	VO
9. Is forgetful in daily activities	N	S	O	VO

Scale B:

	N	S	O	VO
10. Fidgets with hands or feet or squirms in seat	N	S	O	VO
11. Leaves seat in classroom or in other situations when expected to remain seated	N	S	O	VO
12. Runs about or climbs excessively in situations where it is inappropriate (in adolescence, may be limited to restlessness)	N	S	O	VO
13. Has difficulty playing or engaging quietly in leisure activities	N	S	O	VO
14. Is "on the go" or often acts as if "driven by a motor"	N	S	O	VO
15. Talks excessively	N	S	O	VO
16. Blurts out answers before the questions have been completed	N	S	O	VO
17. Has difficulty awaiting turn	N	S	O	VO
18. Interrupts or intrudes on others (eg, butts into others' conversations or games)	N	S	O	VO

Scale C:

	N	S	O	VO
19. Is uncooperative or defiant or argues with adults	N	S	O	VO
20. Has difficulty getting along with other children	N	S	O	VO
21. Is often angry, irritable, or easily upset	N	S	O	VO
22. Has excessive anxiety, worry, or fearfulness	N	S	O	VO
23. Seems sad, moody, depressed, or discouraged	N	S	O	VO
24. Has problems with academic progress (skill level or learning)	N	S	O	VO
25. Has problems with academic performance (productivity or accuracy)	N	S	O	VO

Please comment on this child's strengths, weaknesses, or other concerns on the back of this form.

From Miller KJ, Castellanos FX. Attention deficit hyperactivity disorders. *Pediatr Rev* 1998;19:373.

TABLE 9.2. Differential diagnosis of ADHD

Developmental Differences
  Normal variation
  Cognitive impairment
  Giftedness
  Learning disabilities
  Perceptual/processing disorders
  Language disorders
  Pervasive developmental disorders
  Fragile X syndrome

Medical Disorders
  Sensory impairments
  Seizure disorders
  Sequelae of central nervous system infection/trauma
  Fetal alcohol syndrome
  Lead poisoning
  Iron deficiency anemia
  Neurodegenerative disorders
  Tourette syndrome
  Thyroid disorders
  Substance abuse
  Medication side effect
  Undernutrition
  Sleep disorder

Emotional/Behavioral Disorders
  Depression/Mood disorders
  Anxiety disorders
  Oppositional defiant disorder
  Conduct disorder
  Posttraumatic stress disorder
  Adjustment disorder

Environmental Disorders
  Child abuse/neglect
  Stressful home environment
  Inadequate/punitive parenting
  Parental psychopathology
  Sociocultural difference
  Inappropriate educational setting

Frequently Associated Problems
  Motor coordination disorders
  Social skills deficit
  Enuresis and encopresis

From Miller KJ, Castellanos FX. Attention deficit hyperactivity disorder. *Pediatr Rev* 1998;19:373.

PHYSICAL EXAMINATION

The physical examination is usually normal in the child with ADHD. Particular attention should be paid to the hearing, vision, and neurologic examinations.

LABORATORY EVALUATION

No laboratory tests are recommended for all children with ADHD. Tests that may be indicated include an electroencephalogram, thyroid stimulating hormone, hematocrit, and lead level.

DIAGNOSIS

For diagnosis of ADHD the DSM-IV requires that six of the items in scale A or B of Table 9.1 be "often" or "very often" and to a degree that is maladaptive and inconsistent with developmental level. These behaviors must be present for at least 6 months, and some should be present before 7 years of age. These symptoms should be present in at least two settings (at home, in school, or with peers) and should cause clinically significant impairment. Finally, the symptoms should not be explained by another disorder, although ADHD may be comorbid. Scale C of Table 9.1 lists screening questions for problems commonly associated with ADHD.

MANAGEMENT

The management of ADHD requires a team approach with input from parents; school officials, including the school psychologist; other mental health providers; and the physician. Coordination of this team can be time-consuming, but a coordinated effort is needed for best results. The four main areas of intervention are behavioral, emotional, academic, and pharmacologic. The behavioral aspects of management are best handled through referral to a counselor. Unfortunately, this resource may not always be available. When the family physician must manage the child without this assistance, the parents should be taught to provide increased structure for the child. This may be accomplished by posting family rules and a daily schedule for the child. Parents need to target specific maladaptive behaviors and provide prompt, consistent feedback. Positive reinforcement for good behaviors must not be overlooked. Methods to accomplish this include a point system or sticker chart. Maintaining these interventions is difficult for parents, and they too need positive reinforcement from the physician. Barkley provides many examples of methods of parent training.

Emotional interventions allow the patient and family to cope with the psychologic, social, and family issues that surround ADHD. Support groups can be very beneficial for patients and families. At times, individual, marital, or family therapy may be needed.

Children with ADHD often have academic difficulties. They should be formally evaluated for learning disabilities. School psychologists, when available, can be an invaluable asset. They can test for learning disabilities and help to set up an individualized educational plan. They can also be a source of additional information about the child's school performance both at baseline and with interventions. Children with ADHD may qualify for special educational services under the Individuals with Disabilities Education Act. In the past, children were often "held back," especially in early grades, in the hopes that they would be more mature and so less symptomatic with their ADHD. Recent evidence, however, shows that being old-for-grade, even without being retained, is associated with increased rates of behavior problems, especially among adolescents (Byrd Pediatrics 1997).

TABLE 9.3. Medication for attention deficit/hyperactivity disorder

Medication	Dose	Onset/Duration	Potential Side Effects/Cautions	Follow-up
Pemoline* (Cylert) 18/75, 37.5, 75 mg tablets 37.5 mg chewable	Initial dose, 37.5 mg A.M. Frequency, 1–2 dose/day Must be taken daily Dose range 13.75–112.5 mg/day 2 mg/kg/day	Onset 2 hours Duration 7–10 hours	Life-threatening hepatic failure Insomnia, anorexia, stomachache, headache	Do not use first line Risk of hepatic failure. Monitor serial liver function tests. Informed consent should be obtained (see package insert) Height, weight, blood pressure, pulse
Imipramine (Tofranil) 10, 25, 50 mg	Initial, 10–25 mg at bedtime Frequency, 2–3 doses/day Must be taken daily, stop slowly Dose range, 20–100 mg/day 1–3 mg/kg/day	Maximum effect May take several weeks	May affect cardiac conduction rate Anticholinergic Patients with tics, comorbid anxiety, depression may respond better to tricyclic antidepressants Very dangerous in overdose	Blood pressure, heart rate Consider EKG
Clonidine (Catapres) 0.1, 0.2, 0.3 mg	Initial, 0.05 mg at bedtime Frequency, 3 doses/day Must be taken daily Dose range, 0.1–0.4 mg/day	Maximum effect May take several weeks	Sedation, orthostatic hypotension, depression, nightmares, dizziness, nausea Especially useful with comorbid conduct disorder Very dangerous in overdose Rebound hypertension if stopped abruptly	Monitor blood pressure at baseline and after dose adjustment
Methylphenidate* (MPH) (Ritalin) 5, 10, 20 mg tablets	Initial, 5 mg/dose Frequency, 2–3 doses/day Dose range, 5–80 mg/day 0.3–0.8 mg/kg/dose	Onset, 20–30 minutes Duration, 3–5 hours	Anorexia, insomnia, stomachache Avoid decongestants	Height, weight, blood pressure, pulse, at least yearly

Medication	Dosage	Onset/Duration	Side Effects	Monitoring
Ritalin SR* or generic 20 mg only	Initial, 20 mg Frequency, 1–2 doses/day Dose range, 0.6–2 mg/kg per dose 20–80 mg/day	Onset, 60–90 minutes Duration, 5–8 hours	Anorexia, insomnia, stomachache, headache Avoid decongestants Do not cut or chew tablet	Height, weight, blood pressure, pulse yearly
Dextroamphetamine* (DEX) Dexedrine 5 mg Dextrostat 5, 10 mg	Initial, 2.5–5 mg Frequency, 2–3 doses/day Dose range, 2.5–40 mg/day 0.15–0.4 mg/kg/dose	Onset, 20–60 minutes Duration, 4–6 hours	Anorexia, insomnia, stomachache, headache Avoid decongestants	Height, weight, blood pressure, pulse yearly
Dexedrine spansules* 5, 10, 15 mg	Initial 5 mg in A.M. Frequency, 1–2 doses/day Dose range, 5–40 mg/day 0.3–0.8 mg/kg/dose	Onset, 60–90 minutes Duration, 6–10 hours	Anorexia, insomnia, stomachache, headache Avoid decongestants	Height, weight, blood pressure, pulse yearly

*Approved by FDA for treatment of ADHD.

Adapted from Miller KJ, Castellanos FX. Attention deficit/hyperactivity disorders. Pediatr Rev 1998;19:373; AAP Committee on Children with Disabilities and Committee on Drugs. Medication for children with attentional disorders. Pediatrics 1996;98:301.

Medications are frequently used in the management of ADHD. It must be reemphasized that medications are best used in conjunction with the other treatments mentioned earlier. Also, medications should be used only when the child's ADHD causes difficulties with behavior, school performance, or social adjustment. The mainstays of pharmacologic intervention are the stimulants, especially methylphenidate (Ritalin). The stimulants increase attention span, decrease hyperactivity, and improve impulse control. There has been much debate on the use of sustained-release stimulant preparations. The advantage of these preparations is longer activity, which may make in-school dosing unnecessary. Others claim that the longer-acting preparations are less effective. In reality, because these medications usually show full effect in a couple of weeks, the physician can do a therapeutic trial of the longer-acting medicine. If the child does not do as well on the longer-acting medication, he can be switched back to the immediate release.

Side effects of stimulants are commonly reported, but one study found that these "side effects" are actually preexisting characteristics of children with ADHD and improve with stimulant treatment (Efron, Pediatrics, 1997). In general, stimulants are well tolerated, with the most common side effects being appetite suppression and insomnia. If the stimulants are not effective, other agents such as tricyclic antidepressants or clonidine may be tried. Table 9.3 lists the medications commonly used for ADHD, including dosing and common side effects. Patients may be dosed on evenings, holidays, and weekends if their symptoms interfere with activities during these times.

FOLLOW-UP

Follow-up must be individualized. Monthly visits are often necessary early in the course of treatment, but many patients are seen every 3 months once their condition is stabilized. Approximately annually, a trial off the medication should be done to verify that the medication is still beneficial. Frequently, patients conduct their own trial by, inadvertently or not, forgetting the medication for a period of time. Formal trials may be needed to convince patients, parents, or teachers of benefit. Use of the Conner Scale (Table 9.4) or other symptom-rating scale may allow comparison of a period

T ABLE 9.4.   Conners abbreviated parent-teacher questionnaire

Each item is rated on a scale of 0 to 3. Typical score for hyperactivity is 15 or higher.
1. Restlessness in the "squirming" sense
2. Needs demands met immediately
3. Temper outbursts and unpredictable behavior
4. Distractibility of attention span, which is a problem
5. Disturbs other children
6. Pouts and sulks
7. Quick and drastic mood changes
8. Restlessness—always up and on the go
9. Excitable, impulsive
10. Fails to finish things that he/she starts

Adapted from Goyette CH, Conners CK, Ulrich RF. Normative data on revised Conners Parent and Teacher Rating Scales. *J Abnorm Child Psychol* 1978;6:221.

of time on the medication versus one off the medication. This type of trial is often useful to convince an adolescent patient of the need for continued medication. As children grow, larger doses of medication are usually needed.

REFERRAL

The decision to refer a child with ADHD depends mostly on the personal preference of the physician, the availability of resources in the local community, and the extent of the child's dysfunction. Unfortunately, many of the children with the most severe ADHD may also have social situations that greatly limit their parents' ability to obtain specialized services. These limitations may be financial or, especially in rural areas, related to travel.

REFERENCES

American Academy of Pediatrics Committee on Children with Disabilities and Committee on Drugs. Medication for children with attentional disorder. *Pediatrics* 1996;98:301.

Byrd RS, Weitzman M, Auinger PA. Increased behavior problems associated with delayed school entry and delayed school entry and delayed school progress. *Pediatrics* 1997;100:654.

Efron D, Jarman F, Barker M, Dip G. Side effects of methylphenidate and dexamphetamine in children with attention deficit hyperactivity disorder: a double-blind, crossover trial. *Pediatrics* 1997;100:662.

Lafleur LH, Northup J. ADHD: how school psychologists can help. *Am Fam Physician* 1997;55:773.

Miller KJ, Castellanos FX. Attention deficit/hyperactivity disorders. *Pediatr Rev* 1998;19:373.

Taylor MA. Evaluation and management of attention-deficit hyperactivity disorder. *Am Fam Physician* 1997;55:887.

Physician Resources

Barkley RA. *Attention-deficit hyperactivity disorder: a handbook for diagnosis and treatment.* New York: Guilford Press, 1990.

Conners CK. Conners Rating Scales-Revised (1997). Multi-Health Systems, 908 Niagara Falls Boulevard, North Tonowanda, NY 14120. 800-456-3003.

Gordon M, Irwin, M. *The diagnosis and treatment of ADD/ADHD: a no nonsense guide for primary care physicians.* Dewitt, NY: GSI Publications, 1997. 800-550-ADHD. Includes computer diskette with reproducible forms.

Patient Education/Resources

ADD Warehouse. www.addwarehouse.com. Large selection of titles for parents and children with ADHD.

ADHD: Does my child have it? Handout available from AAFP online at www.familydoctor.org.

ADHD medicine. Handout available from AAFP online at www.familydoctor.org.

Barkley RA. *Taking charge of AD/HD: the complete guide for parents.* New York: Guilford Press, 1995. 800-365-7006.

Children and Adults with Attention Deficit-Hyperactivity Disorder. www.CHADD.org. Largest support organization for children and adults with ADHD.

Books for Children

Gavin M. *Otto learns about his medicine: a story about medication for hyperactive children.* New York: Magination Press, 1995.

Moss DM. Shelley the hyperactive turtle. Kensington, MD: Woodbine House 1989.

Anorexia and Bulimia
by Gregory B. Mack and Jeanne M. Spencer

Anorexia and bulimia typically affect 1% to 5% of adolescent girls and young women. Although most cases occur in females, approximately 10% occur in males. The mortality rate from anorexia is unacceptably high, at 0.56% per year, which is 12 times as high as the mortality rate among young women in the general population. The mortality rate reaches 8% at a mean of 5 years and up to 20% in cases of chronic anorexia or bulimia. The causes of death are varied, but are most commonly suicide, infection, and effects of electrolyte disturbance, including cardiac arrhythmia and sudden death. Currently, only about half of patients with anorexia or bulimia experience a full recovery, 30% recover partially, and 20% show no substantial improvement. Despite improvement in the treatment of these disorders, treatment failures and substantial delays in diagnosis persist. A multidisciplinary approach to treatment that includes medical, nutritional, and psychologic professionals is usually most effective. Family physicians can play an essential role in the treatment team, especially in facilitating diagnosis and long-term follow-up.

HISTORY

Rarely does the patient recognize the condition herself. In fact, the disorder cannot really exist without denial. Typically, the patient's parents seek medical attention for their daughter because of her low body weight, fatigue, depression, isolation, or amenorrhea. Most patients have already reached a body mass index of 15% below ideal at presentation. Parents may be aware of the child's vomiting, use of laxatives, or exercise with a goal of weight reduction. The patient may be reluctant to give a history, but the following questions (in either written or verbal form) may facilitate discussion:

Do you feel sick when you sit down at the table?

Are you afraid to touch any foods?

Do you eat your foods in a certain order?

Do you have a different view of your body from that of other people?

Do you prefer to eat by yourself?

Do your family or friends "bug" you about what you eat?

Does anyone tell you that you spend too much time in physical activity?

Do you get upset if something isn't perfect?

Do you tear your food into tiny pieces before eating it?

Are you overly afraid to be seen in public in a swimsuit?

Do you avoid certain foods because you think they are going to change the way you look?

If possible, the physician should obtain a detailed history of caloric intake, purging activities (including vomiting and laxative use), exercise, and weight loss.

FAMILY HISTORY

A family history of depression or obsessive-compulsive disorder is often present, and sometimes one or both parents meet the criteria for an eating disorder. The family history often reveals multiple stressors or trauma. Physical and sexual abuse are more common in patients with bulimia than in the general population.

SOCIAL HISTORY

Patients often live in dual-income, professional families. Frequently the child is involved in multiple activities such as ballet, gymnastics, track, or soccer and is remarkable for her leadership, compassion, or academic success. Males are often wrestlers. Patients rarely engage in typical adolescent activities such as dating or attending parties. Often the patient has been placed in a caretaker role within her family. Anorexia frequently presents in early high school at the time of menarche. Bulimia often presents during the first semester in college.

PHYSICAL EXAMINATION

Accurately measuring height and weight is essential. Care must be taken to ensure that the patient is not falsifying the weight. Weighing the child facing away from the scale may reduce anxiety. Table 9.5 lists the typical physical findings and medical complications in anorexic and bulimic patients. The body mass index (BMI) is calculated by dividing the weight in kilograms (divide weight in pounds by 2.2 lb/kg) by the square of the height in meters (divide height in inches by 39.37 in./m).

Ideal body weight is generally estimated as follows:

$$\text{BMI} = 20 \text{ for age over } 16$$
$$\text{BMI} = 18.5 - 19.5 \text{ for age } 14 \text{ to } 15$$

Below age 14 a standard growth chart is used.

LABORATORY EVALUATION

Table 9.6 lists the usual initial laboratory evaluation of the patient with an eating disorder.

Initially normal laboratory results may be falsely reassuring because electrolyte abnormalities frequently occur with refeeding.

An EKG should be obtained as soon as possible, mainly for the purpose of calculating the QT_c interval (see Chapter 7, Fig. 7.2). If the QT_c interval is more than 0.45, the patient is at risk for ventricular tachycardia. In itself a QT_c of 0.5 or greater usually necessitates hospital admission for cardiac monitoring. With refeeding, electrolyte shifts can quickly prolong the QT_c.

DIFFERENTIAL DIAGNOSIS

The differential diagnosis for severe anorexia is long and can include hypothalamic tumor, hypoadrenalism, hyperthyroidism, immunocompromised states, severe

T ABLE 9.5. Physical findings/medical complications and laboratory abnormalities of anorexia nervosa and bulimia nervosa

System	Eating Disorder	
	Anorexia	**Bulimia**
Cardiovascular	Dilated cardiomyopathy	Arrhythmias
	Arrhythmias (premature ventricular contractions, bradycardia, ventricular tachycardia, atrial fibrillation)	Ipecac-induced cardiopathy
	EKG changes (prolonged QT_c, T-wave changes, etc.)	Hypotension
	Myocardial infarctions	
	Refeeding edema	
	Hypotension	
Hematologic	Leukopenia	Increased bleeding tendencies
	Lymphocytosis	
	Neutropenia	
	Bleeding diathesis secondary to prolonged bleeding time, prolonged PT, or prolonged PTT	
	Bone marrow hypocellularity	
	Impaired immune function	
	Anemia	
Pulmonary	Subcutaneous emphysema	Aspiration pneumonitis from self-induced vomiting
Dermatologic	Hair loss	Finger calluses/abrasions (Russell's sign)
		Clubbing

Metabolic	Lanugo-like hair growth	Hypokalemia
	Dry skin, brittle hair and nails	Hyponatremia
	Petechiae, purpura (thrombocytopenia)	Hypochloremia
	Yellowing of skin (hypercarotenemia)	Hypomagnesemia
	Impaired taste	Hypocalcemia
	Hypercholesterolemia	Hyperuricemia
	Hypercarotinemia	Increased amylase level
	Zinc deficiency	Metabolic alkalosis
	Abnormal liver function tests	
	Abnormal glucose tolerance	
	Fasting hypoglycemia	
	Hypocalcemia (tetany)	
	Hypothermia	
Gastrointestinal	Altered gastric emptying	Bloating
	Salivary gland swelling	Constipation
	Superior mesenteric artery syndrome	Increased amylase level
	Gastric dilatation	Delayed gastric emptying
	Constipation	Reflux esophagitis
	Parotid gland swelling	Gastric rupture
	Pancreatic dysfunction	Parotid gland swelling
		Cathartic colon (megacolon)
		Malabsorption syndrome

continued

TABLE 9.5. Physical findings/medical complications and laboratory abnormalities of anorexia nervosa and bulimia nervosa *(continued)*

System	Eating Disorder	
	Anorexia	**Bulimia**
Laxative complications		
Renal	Dehydration	Dehydration
	Elevated blood urea nitrogen	Elevated blood urea nitrogen
	Decreased renal function	Decreased glomerular filtration rate
	Kaliopenic nephropathy	Urinary concentrating defect
Endocrine	Amenorrhea/oligomenorrhea	Blunted thyroid-stimulating hormone response to thyroid-releasing hormone
	Decreased hypothalamic activity	Pathologic growth hormone response to TRH/glucose
	Decreased estrogen	Prolactin elevations
	Decreased testosterone	Abnormal dexamethasone suppression test (nonsuppression)
	Hypothyroidism	Osteomalacia
	Increased growth hormone	
	Increased cortisol	
	Abnormal dexamethasone suppression test	
	Osteoporosis	
	Delayed puberty	

Central Nervous System	Cortical atrophy Ventricular dilation Cognitive impairment EEG abnormalities Depression Hyperactivity Neuropathy	EEG abnormalities (64%) Depression
Dental problems	Decalcification Caries	Caries Enamel erosion

T ABLE 9.6. Initial labs

Glucose, sodium, potassium, blood urea nitrogen, creatinine, magnesium, zinc, phosphorus
CBC with differential
Free T4, Thyroid-stimulating hormone (TSH)
Urinalysis
Liver function tests
Cholesterol, triglyceride, high-density lipoprotein, low-density lipoprotein
Other tests that are especially useful in documenting the degree of malnutrition:
    Serum iron, ferritin
    Total complement

T ABLE 9.7. Diagnostic criteria for eating disorders

Anorexia nervosa
Body weight <85% of expected weight (or body-mass index ≤17.5)
Intense fear of weight gain
Inaccurate perception of own body size, weight, or shape
Amenorrhea (in girls and women after menarche)
Bulimia nervosa
Recurrent binge eating (at least two times per week for three months)*
Recurrent purging, excessive exercise, or fasting (at least two times per week for three months)
Excessive concern about body weight or shape
Absence of anorexia nervosa
Binge-eating disorder
Recurrent binge eating (at least two days per week for six months)*
Marked distress with at least three of the following:
    Eating very rapidly
    Eating until uncomfortably full
    Eating when not hungry
    Eating alone
    Feeling disgusted or guilty after a binge
No recurrent purging, excessive exercise, or fasting
Absence of anorexia nervosa
Other (atypical) eating disorders
Clinically important disordered eating, inappropriate weight control, or excessive concern about body weight or
    shape that does not meet all the criteria for anorexia nervosa, bulimia nervosa, or binge-eating disorder

*A binge is characterized by the consumption of an unusually large quantity of food during a discrete period of
time, with lack of control over eating.

Adapted from the *Diagnostic and Statistical Manual of Mental Disorders,* 4th ed. Washington, D.C.: American
Psychiatric Association, 1995; and Becker AE, et al. Eating disorders. *N Eng J Med* 1999;340:1092.

depression, chronic infection, inflammatory bowel disease, and underlying carcinoma. In patients with any of the preceding causes of anorexia, one can usually find a supportive historic or physical finding and one does not find the distorted thinking patterns pertaining to food and weight. Table 9.7 lists the diagnostic criteria for eating disorders.

MANAGEMENT

Caution is needed in refeeding the patient who has severe malnutrition. Rapid shifts of electrolytes are possible and can lead to arrhythmias. If refeeding is done on an outpatient basis, electrolytes should be closely monitored, especially if the patient had been using excessive purging or water intake. Table 9.8 lists criteria for in patient admission.

In a severely malnourished patient receiving inpatient treatment, refeeding syndrome should be anticipated even if electrolytes are initially normal. In this syndrome, rapid shifts of electrolytes may lead to dysrhythmias. Patients should be on a cardiac monitor, and if renal function is normal and the electrolytes are normal, started on one-half normal saline with 20 to 40 mEq/L of K-phos (without dextrose or oral feedings). The intravenous (IV) fluids need to be altered to compensate for abnormalities that were present at the onset of treatment or that occur during treatment. If the electrolytes are stable after 24 hours of IV fluids, oral intake may be encouraged and D5 may be added to the IV fluids.

Nutritional education is essential and is usually carried out by a dietitian. For anorexia nervosa, weight gain is one of the primary goals; therefore patients need to be educated on caloric requirements and expenditures. Generally, patients begin with

TABLE 9.8. Criteria for inpatient treatment for eating disorders

Medical instability (e.g., hypokalemia, renal failure, congestive heart failure, prolonged QT_c)
Weight loss of greater than 20% of ideal body weight
Unresponsive to outpatient care
Comorbid psychiatric conditions (e.g., schizophrenia, suicidal ideation, substance abuse, and mania)
Dysfunctional family system
Treatment resistance
Weight change of 20 lb (9 kg) or more within the past 4 months
Caloric intake of 700 or less a day
Fasting 3 or more consecutive days each week for 4 weeks
Refusing prescribed electrolyte treatment
Refusing prescribed treatment for medical problems
Frequent fainting spells
Confirmed diagnosis of a heart condition related to the eating disorder
Binging more than seven times per week
Binging on excessively large quantities of food
Self-induced vomiting several times a day
Laxative and diuretic abuse on a daily basis
Multiple hours of daily exercise
Ipecac use regardless of the frequency

a diet consisting of their previous intake plus 200 calories per day. This is usually distributed between three meals and three snacks. The amount of calories can be increased every 3 to 5 days. Initially, the goal is weight stabilization, followed by a gain of 0.25 to 0.5 pound per week. A multivitamin and calcium at 1,000 to 1,500 mg/day is recommended to reduce the osteopenia in anorexia nervosa. Goal weight or ideal weight is typically a BMI of 20; this is lower in younger children (see earlier).

In anorexia, a combination of individual, group, and family therapy is most effective. Cognitive behavioral therapy and interpersonal psychotherapy are effective for bulimia. If the patient is severely malnourished, cognitive deficits may limit therapy until weight gain occurs.

The use of antidepressant drugs has become routine in the treatment of anorexia and bulimia, particularly the selective serotonin reuptake inhibitors (SSRIs). Fluoxetine (Prozac) has been the most studied in the treatment of anorexia and appears to have an effect in those patients with severe depression. The effect of the SSRIs will be inhibited or limited until nutrition is restored to reasonable levels. SSRIs are also very effective in the treatment of bulimia. In bulimic patients who do not respond to SSRIs, venlafaxine (Effexor), which is a potent reuptake inhibitor of serotonin and norepinephrine and a weak reuptake inhibitor of dopamine, may be effective.

Families play a key role in treatment. Often the illness has caused great stress for the family members, who may feel guilty about the illness. Once these issues are addressed, the family can begin to participate in the treatment of the child. Family therapy may be very beneficial, even in families that appear "normal" on the surface.

REFERRAL

Programs for the treatment of eating disorders vary widely in their treatment approach and efficacy. Table 9.9 lists characteristics of successful programs.

FOLLOW-UP

Patients should be seen at least weekly at the onset. These visits should include measuring weight, if the weight is not followed elsewhere. As the patient improves, the frequency of visits may be decreased, especially if the patient is attending counseling or sessions with the dietitian.

Patients who have completed an in-patient program frequently return to the family physician's medical care. These patients need close follow-up, especially as they readjust to home and school life. During this time they should follow up with the dietitian, and participate in individual, group, and family therapy. Because eating disorders are chronic conditions, patients should be followed closely for at least the first 2 years after diagnosis.

REFERENCES

Becker AE, Grinspoon SK, Klibanski A, Herzog DB. Eating disorders. *N Engl J Med* 1999;340:1092.

Beumont PJ, Large M. Hypophosphataemia, delirium and cardiac arrhythmia in anorexia nervosa. *Med J Aust* 1991;155:519.

Birmingham CL, Alothman AF, Goldner EM. Anorexia nervosa: refeeding and hypophosphatemia. *Int J Eat Disord* 1996;20:211.

Hobbs WL, Johnson CA. Anorexia nervosa: an overview. *Am Fam Physician* 1996;54:1273.

T ABLE 9.9. Characteristics of successful treatment programs for eating disorders

Outpatient treatment
  Team approach, including
  Medical
  Nutritional
  Psychiatric
  Psychologic
  Individual therapy
  Family therapy
  Group therapy for families and patients
Inpatient treatment
  At least 40 hours of organized time per week
  On-staff medical coverage
  Staff treats only eating disorders
  Population restricted to patients with eating disorders
  Individual therapy
  Process group therapy
  Didactic group therapy
  Psychodrama
  Nutrition classes
  Academic services (continuation of academic studies)
  Spiritual growth groups
  Extensive family therapy
  Activities therapy (e.g., art therapy, body image therapy, leisure activity planning)
  Relapse prevention
  Special attention to issues of:
    Addiction
    Codependency
    Sexual abuse
    Depression
    Life skills
  Aftercare follow-up and planning
  Predetermined payment and contractual agreement for at least 45 days of inpatient treatment

Kohn MR, Golden NH, Shenker IR. Cardiac arrest and delirium: presentations of the refeeding syndrome in severely malnourished adolescents with anorexia nervosa. *J Adolesc Health* 1998;22:239.

McGilley B, Pryor TL. Assessment and treatment of bulimia nervosa. *Am Fam Physician* 1998;57:2743.

Moukaddem M, Boulier A, Apfelbaum M, Rigaud D. Increase in diet-induced thermogenesis at the start of refeeding in severely malnourished anorexia nervosa patients. *Am J Clin Nutr* 1997;66:133.

Worley G, Claerhout SJ, Combs SP. Hypophosphatemia in malnourished children during refeeding. *Clin Pediatr* 1998;37:347.

Patient Education/Resources

Anorexia Nervosa and Related Eating Disorders, Inc. 541-344-1144. www.anred.com. Clearinghouse of information.

Anorexia nervosa. Handout available from AAFP online at www.familydoctor.org.

Remuda Ranch. 800-445-1900. www.remuda-ranch.com. Inpatient and outpatient treatment, patient education.

Vredevelt P, Newman D, Beverly H, Minirith F. *Thin disguise.* Nashville: Nelsonword Publishing Group, 1996.

Professional Resources

Academy for Eating Disorders. 703-556-9222. www.acadeatdis.org. Patient and professional education.

Garner DM, Garfinkel PE. *Handbook for the treatment of eating disorders,* 2nd ed. New York: Guilford Press, 1997.

International Association for Eating Disorder Professionals. 407-831-7099. Certifies professionals who specialize in eating disorders.

Depression

CHIEF COMPLAINT

"I think something is wrong with my child." "I think my child is depressed."

HISTORY OF PRESENT ILLNESS

The history is the most important element in the evaluation of the potentially depressed child. Depression presents differently, depending on the age of the child. Depression in infancy and early childhood is difficult to detect. These children may present with persistent apathy, despondency, nonorganic failure to thrive, and sleep difficulties. School-aged children can begin to express a feeling of sadness. They may have a loss of interest and pleasure from activities and may have low self-esteem, describing themselves as bad, stupid, or ugly. Chronic fatigue, irritability, guilt, somatic complaints, and social withdrawal are common. Depressed adolescents have more apparent loss of interest and pleasure, hypersomnia, feeling of hopelessness, and weight change than younger children. They may have difficulty interacting in peer groups. Table 9.10 lists helpful questions to ask in taking the history. Suicidality must be assessed. Children are at imminent risk if they have an identified plan with access to lethal means, a history of recent or recurrent suicide attempts, severe depression, psychotic symptoms, or substance abuse.

PAST MEDICAL HISTORY

Depression is more common in children with chronic medical illness. Comorbidity is common with anxiety, conduct and oppositional defiant disorder, and ADHD.

TABLE 9.10.   Psychosocial questions for use with children and caregivers

Questions for Parents

Have there been any changes in your family or life-style?

How do you and your spouse work together in raising your child?

How do you handle disagreements in raising your children or between yourselves?

Has your family ever been through a major crisis? How did you cope?

Have you or any of the members of your family ever suffered from a mental illness or substance abuse
    problem? Are you aware of any effect that this problem may have had on your child?

What emotions do you see in your child these days?

Has your child suffered the loss of someone important to him or her?

Do you think your child is drinking alcohol or using drugs?

Has your teenager (or child) ever tried to hurt himself or herself intentionally?

Questions for Children

Everyone feels sad or angry at times. How about you?

Do you feel sad almost every day . . . most of the time?

What makes you feel that bad?

Did you ever feel so upset that you wished you were not alive or that you wanted to die?

Did you ever do something so dangerous that you could have gotten hurt or killed?

Did you ever intentionally try to kill yourself?

Used with permission from Hack S, Jellinek M. Historical clues to the diagnosis of the dysfunctional child and other psychiatric disorders in children. *Pediatr Clin North Am* 1998;45:25.

FAMILY HISTORY

Depression is more common in children whose parents have had depression.

SOCIAL HISTORY

Families with depressed children often have difficulty with communication, emotional support, and conflict resolution. Parental dysfunction, divorce, and child abuse may be present. Parents may be coping with their own mental illness. In both the patient and the family, the abuse of substances, including alcohol, should be assessed.

PHYSICAL EXAMINATION

Determining the need for other testing to rule out organic causes of the symptoms is the most important role for the physical examination. Particular attention should be paid to signs of physical abuse, adenopathy (malignancy), and the neurologic examination.

LABORATORY EVALUATION

Screening laboratory tests may include complete blood count, electrolytes, blood urea nitrogen, creatinine, liver function tests, and thyroid function tests, directed by the history and physical examination findings.

DIAGNOSIS

Table 9.11 lists the DSM-IV criteria for the Diagnosis of Depression; Table 9.12 lists medical conditions that may mimic depression; and Table 9.13 lists the psychiatric differential diagnosis.

MANAGEMENT

Suicidal children need psychiatric consultation. If the child is at imminent suicidal risk, hospitalization may be necessary. Psychotherapy, especially with a cognitive behavioral approach, is often beneficial. Once an extensive evaluation is completed, the family physician can often comanage the patient, with most of the visits occurring in the family practice setting. The frequency of follow-up visits can be determined jointly by the patient, family, psychiatrist or psychologist, and family physician. A long-standing relationship with the patient and family can facilitate long-term intervention. Serotonin reuptake inhibitors (SSRIs) are the mainstay of treatment of depression in children (Table 9.14). They may be started at initial diagnosis or after a trial of psychotherapy alone. In general, the dose is increased only every 4 to 6 weeks, using the "start low, go slow" philosophy. Common side effects include sedation, activation (meaning "increased activity"), or gastrointestinal side effects. Tricyclic antidepressants have not been proved to be effective in childhood depression. Support groups for both the child and the parents may be helpful.

FOLLOW-UP

Follow-up of the depressed child depends on the individual situation, including severity of illness and involvement of other care providers. Early in treatment the child may be seen weekly, with visit intervals extended in those patients being seen by multiple providers. Generally, medication should be continued for a number of months after

T ABLE 9.11. **DSM IV criteria for major depressive episode**

Five of the following symptoms have been present during the same 2-week period and represent a change from previous functioning; at least one of the symptoms is either depressed mood or loss of interest or pleasure.
   Depressed mood or irritable mood
   Markedly diminished interest or pleasure in activities
   Significant weight change or appetite disturbance
   Insomnia or hypersomnia
   Psychomotor agitation or retardation
   Fatigue or loss of energy
   Feelings of worthlessness or guilt
   Disturbed concentration or indecisiveness
   Recurrent thoughts of death, suicidal ideation, or suicide attempt

T ABLE 9.12. Conditions mimicking depression in children and adolescents

Infections	Neuro/tumor	Endocrine
Mononucleosis	Epilepsy	Diabetes
Influenza	Postconcussion	Cushing disease
Encephalitis	Subarachnoid hemorrhage	Addison disease
Pneumonia	Cerebrovascular accident	Hypothyroidism
Tuberculosis	Multiple sclerosis	Hyperthyroidism
Hepatitis	Huntington disease	Hyperparathyroidism
Syphilis		Hypopituitarism
AIDS		

Medications	Others
Antihypertensives	Alcohol and drug abuse (drug abuse and withdrawal)
Barbiturates	Cocaine
Benzodiazepines	Amphetamine
Corticosteroids	Opiates
Oral contraceptives	Electrolyte abnormality
Cimetidine (Tagamet)	Hypokalemia
Aminophylline	Hyponatremia
Anticonvulsants	Failure to thrive
Clonidine (Catapres)	Anemia
Digitalis	Lupus
Thiazide diuretics	Wilson disease
	Porphyria
	Uremia

Used with permission from Wise MG, Rundell JR. *Concise Guide to Consultation Psychiatry.* Washington, DC: American Psychiatric Press; 1988.

cessation of symptoms. If the symptoms recur, prolonged treatment is indicated. Specialist referral may be needed if the initial treatment is ineffective. SSRIs should be gradually tapered, as abrupt discontinuation can lead to withdrawl symptoms, which include dizziness, headache, nausea, headache, sensory disturbances, and mood disturbance.

T ABLE 9.13. Psychiatric differential diagnosis of depression in children

Adjustment disorder: Depressive symptoms do not fulfill the criteria for depression
Uncomplicated bereavement: Symptoms must persist beyond 2 months for depression
Separation anxiety disorder: Symptoms are only present when separated from a loved one
Bipolar disorder: Mania in children may present with irritability instead of euphoria.
ADD is less likely if the attention span was normal before the depression

T ABLE 9.14. Pediatric dosing and costs of SSRIs

SSRI	Pediatric Dosage (qd)	Preparations		AWP (100 count)
Fluoxetine (Prozac)	5–40 mg (60 mg) q A.M.	Capsule:	10 mg	$235.63
			20 mg	$241.68
		Oral suspension:	20 mg/5 mL	$107.34/120 mL
Sertraline (Zoloft)	25–125 mg (150 mg) q A.M.	Tablet:	25 mg†,§	$208.76
			50 mg§	$215.55
			100 mg§	$221.79
Paroxetine (Paxil)	5–40 mg (60 mg) q A.M.	Tablet:	10 mg‡	$205.53
			20 mg§	$214.76
			30 mg‡	$220.61
			40 mg‡	$233.13

Reprinted with permission from Labellarte MJ, Walkup JT, Riddle MA. The new antidepressants: selective serotonin reuptake inhibitors. *Pediatr Clin North Am* 1998;45:1137. SSRI, selective serotonin reuptake inhibitor.

Dose range is for preadolescents. Dose = upper limits for adolescent. AWP, average wholesale price.

*McKesson Drug Company, July 7, 1998.

†Available only in 50-count.

‡Available only in 30-count.

§Scored tablet.

REFERRAL

In general, depressed children should be referred for specialist evaluation. The referral resources will vary from community to community, and, more recently, with insurance coverage. Family physicians may need to advocate for patients to get the specialized care they need.

REFERENCES

The Classification of Child and Adolescent Mental Diagnoses in Primary Care. Diagnostic and Statistical Manual for Primary Care (DSM-PC), Child and Adolescent Version. Elk Grove Village, IL: AAP, 1996.

Jellinek MS, Snyder JB. Depression and suicide in children and adolescents. *Pediatr Rev* 1998;19:255.

Labellarte MJ, Walkup JT, Riddle MA. The new antidepressants: selective serotonin reuptake inhibitors. *Pediatr Clin North Am* 1998;45:1137.

McConville BJ, et al. Newer antidepressants: beyond selective serotonin reuptake inhibitors. *Pediatr Clin North Am* 1998;45:1157.

Patient Education/Resources

Dubuque N, Dubuque S. Kid power: tactics for dealing with depression. 1996.

Dubuque S. A parent's survival guide to childhood depression. King of Prussia: Center for Applied Psychology, Inc., 1996.

Dumas LS, Fassler DG. *Help me, I'm sad: recognizing and treating childhood depression.* New York: Viking Press, 1997.

Physician Resources

Findling RL, Blumer JL. eds. Child and adolescent psychopharmacology. *Pediatr Clin North Am*, 1998;45:1. Includes chapters on depression, ADHD, mood stabilizers, all including pediatric dosing.

CHAPTER 10
....

Special Social Situations

Foster Children

Children in foster care are some of the neediest patients seen by the family physician. They have often been exposed to physical, sexual, or mental abuse. Increasingly, they come from homes damaged by the effects of substance abuse. Foster families are usually warm, caring, and altruistic, with a keen desire to help children. Yet some are not and may be harmful to the children in their care. The foster care system is overburdened with increasing numbers of children, decreased funding, and especially in large urban areas, a severe lack of qualified foster families. Kindred care, or care by extended family members, usually grandmothers or aunts, is becoming increasingly common. Potential benefits include maintenance of the ethnic and family ties. Potential hazards include overburdening often impoverished, elderly caregivers. Also, if the child rearing within the family had been suboptimal in the past, this may persist with kindred care. Studies are needed to evaluate the outcomes of kindred care. Family physicians who care for these children can assist foster parents and case workers to maximize the potential for good outcomes for these children.

HISTORY

Obtaining a history on a foster child can be one of the most frustrating aspects of the evaluation. Usually the child presents with a foster parent who has only known the child for a short time and is unaware of his or her medical history. The child may be understandably anxious about disclosing previous injuries and may be unaware of past medical problems. Medical records from previous providers are usually obtainable through parental consent or court order, but this process may be time-consuming. At times past records are unrevealing, as the child may have received only brief care from that provider. Mental health records are most difficult to obtain. Except in the very young child, the child should be interviewed in part away from adult caregivers, to allow the child to express concerns with the current situation. Multiple encounters may be needed before the child shares more sensitive information.

DEVELOPMENT

Developmental assessment is essential for the preschool child. As more than half of foster children are developmentally delayed, the physician should have a low threshold for referral for a comprehensive evaluation. Common developmental disorders include delayed speech and language, fine motor difficulties, and educational disorders. Preschool or school records may be helpful if available. In school-aged children, developmental assessment, including physical and educational, may be obtained through the school.

SOCIAL HISTORY

The physician should be aware of the members of the household. Often foster families bring foster children to their own family physician, and so, the parents and the physician may be well acquainted. The case worker or foster family should be able to outline the reason for placement. The physician should be aware of the interaction with the biologic family, including the extended family, and the anticipated duration and expected outcome of placement. As these plans change frequently, they should be reviewed at subsequent visits.

PHYSICAL EXAMINATION

The child should be examined disrobed so that any physical signs of abuse can be detected. Especially with the previously abused child, adequate chaperoning is essential, both to minimize the child's fears when disrobed with an unfamiliar adult and to limit allegations against the physician. As physical ailments are much more common in this population and the history is likely to be incomplete, the examination should be especially detailed. Areas of particular attention include the skin; heart, for murmurs; lungs, for wheezing; and genitals, for signs of infection and trauma. A neurologic examination should also be done. Age-appropriate hearing and visual screening should be completed.

MEDICAL HEALTH

Children in foster care have a high frequency of medical ailments. Table 10.1 lists conditions most common in foster children.

Management of any of these is complicated by the foster care placement. The physician will need to gauge treatment based on estimates of the expected duration of placement. Foster parents vary widely in their medical knowledge. For example, some may easily handle a difficult asthmatic, whereas with others this may necessitate a placement change. Clear, written instructions may facilitate compliance.

T ABLE 10.1. Common medical conditions in foster children

Respiratory problems (asthma)
Iron deficiency anemia
Failure to thrive
Hearing problems
Recurrent otitis media
Short stature
Enuresis
Encoporesis
Dental caries, malocclusion
Visual problems
Neurologic problems—seizures, fine motor delay

MENTAL HEALTH

Foster children have overwhelming mental health needs. Some may be receiving multiple psychotropic medications with little documentation of previous psychiatric evaluation. Unfortunately, in some cases medications have been used in an attempt to overcome the effects of poor parenting. In nearly all cases the child should be referred for counseling and/or psychiatric evaluation. Mental disorders may result from emotional upheaval, especially with multiple placements, inadequate parenting, prenatal substance exposure, and poor nutrition.

HEALTH MAINTENANCE

Many foster children have not had preventive medical care. Immunization records are often most readily available from the previous school. In young children they may be very difficult to obtain. Immunizations should be given at the first opportunity, as these children may not remain in care for subsequent follow-up. Screening for tuberculosis, HIV, anemia, and hepatitis is usually indicated.

LEGAL ISSUES

Complex legal issues surround the medical care of foster children. In most cases the biologic parents retain legal custody and must give consent for medical care. In many instances foster parents may give consent for routine care, whereas parental consent or a court order may be needed for invasive procedures. Consent for HIV testing varies from state to state and should be clarified before testing. Confidentiality may be very confusing, especially for adolescents.

FINANCIAL

Foster parents are usually provided a daily stipend that covers the child's room, board, and recreation. The amount generally varies from $300 to $1,000 per month, with the higher reimbursement for the most needy children. Travel and clothing expenses are often reimbursed. Foster children are generally eligible for Medicaid and Early and Periodic Screening Diagnosis and Treatment (EPSDT), although coverage is often delayed, particularly with kindred care. Because of the small monthly stipend, most foster parents are unable to provide for medical care not covered by the child's insurance.

ADVOCACY

Foster parents take on the burden of highly needy children, usually with minimal financial compensation beyond expenses. Family physicians should recognize their efforts and support them. Often the physician is able to guide the foster parent toward community resources or empower the foster parents in their interactions with the complex bureaucracy. As community leaders, family physicians should make political leaders aware of the need to fund foster care adequately and to seek its improvement constantly.

REFERENCES

Committee on Early Childhood, Adoption, and Dependent Care. American Academy of Pediatrics. Developmental issues in foster care for children. *Pediatrics* 1993;91:1007.

Gitlitz B, Kuehne E. Caring for children in foster care. *J Pediatr Health Care* 1997;11: 127.

Nordhaus BF, Solnit AJ. Foster placement. *Child Adolesc Psychiatr Clin N Am* 1998;7: 345.

Simms MD. Medical care of children who are homeless or in foster care. *Curr Opin Pediatr* 1998;10:486.

Szilagyi M. The pediatrician and the child in foster care. *Pediatr Rev* 1998;19:39.

Patient Resources
The Foster Parent Pages. www.fostercare.org.

Teenage Mothers

In the United States, approximately 500,000 babies are born to teenage mothers each year, and 25% of women in the United States become pregnant before the age of 18. These mothers experience the additional stress of progressing through their own adolescent development while parenting. Some teen mothers adapt very well to the stressors of parenting; others need extra assistance. Longstanding relationships often make family physicians ideally situated to assist these families. Visits for mother, child, and often grandparents can be used to continually assess the home situation and offer guidance.

Teenage mothers vary in their socioeconomic and social status. For some families a teen pregnancy is expected; in others it is a source of shame. The reaction of the family will greatly affect the teen's level of support, both financial and emotional. Important questions to ask during the pregnancy and well-child visits include the following:

1. How do you feel about parenthood?
2. Is the child's father involved? If so, in what way?
3. How are your friends treating you?
4. How are your parents reacting to the new grandchild?
5. Where are you living?
6. What are your plans for school and work?
7. What child care arrangements have you made?
8. Do you get any time for yourself?

Adolescents may be reluctant to open up at first, but they often accept advice from a respected physician sooner than from parents. Accentuating the strengths of the teen's parenting may help strengthen the bond between provider and patient, and may bolster the teen's self-esteem. Some common strengths of teen parents include physical stamina, optimism, adaptability, and strong peer and family networks.

Table 10.2 lists issues that commonly arise at specific developmental stages of the infant.

While coping with the demands of parenting, the teen must also complete her own development. Young teens especially may have issues about their own body development. The demands of parenting may leave little time for the parent to develop peer relationships, establish an adult relationship with her own parents, complete her education, or choose a career. Teen parents may not have developed their own operational thinking yet, as this commonly occurs between the ages of 10 and 18 years. Without this ability they may be unable to predict the likely consequences

T ABLE 10.2. Common issues for teen mothers during child's development

Newborn	Physical recovery
	Adapting to maternal role and responsibilities
	Three-generation family
Infant	Return to school or work
	Child care
	Relationship with child's father
Toddler	Loss of perceived unconditional love from infant
	Mother and child moving out on own
	Learning to discipline child
	Mother's impulse control during "terrible 2's"
School age	Child's behavioral and learning problems
Adolescence	Loss of teen mother's own childhood
	Frustration over child repeating parent's "mistakes"

Adapted from Kohlenberg TM. Teen mothers. In: Parker S, Zuckerman B, eds. Behavioral and developmental pediatrics. Boston: Little, Brown, 1995:396.

of their actions or weigh alternatives. This cognitive immaturity may lead to risk-taking behavior, such as unprotected sexual intercourse, and may hinder parenting.

Most studies have found that teen parents are just as warm as older counterparts, but they tend to be less verbal, sensitive, responsive, and more authoritarian, and to have unrealistic expectations for their child's development. Whether these findings are due to the age of the parent compared with socioeconomic status is debated. Nevertheless, during the office visits the physician can address these potential deficits. The physician should be aware that the cognitive and behavioral function of the children of teen parents tends to decline as they age; therefore these areas should be explored as the child grows older.

Depending on the level and quality of support and the mother's own abilities, she may benefit from early intervention programs, peer support groups, or parenting classes. Teen parents often ask fewer questions at well-child visits than most new parents. The physician should try to ascertain how things are really going at home and what questions have been left unasked. At times specific inquiry, such as how do you prepare the bottles or what do you do when the child is fussy, may be helpful. More frequent office visits than with older parents may be needed.

Up to half of teen mothers become pregnant again. The desire for other children should be assessed. If another pregnancy is not planned, contraception should be discussed immediately post partum and followed up frequently at subsequent visits. Risk factors for rapid repeat pregnancy include low socioeconomic status, low maternal education, intended first pregnancy, and marriage (Rigsby).

REFERENCES

Coley RL, Chase-Lindale PL. Adolescent pregnancy and parenthood: recent evidence and future directions. *Am Psychol* 1998;53:152.

Kohlenberg TM. Teen mothers. In: Parker S, Zuckerman B, eds. *Behavioral and developmental pediatrics.* Boston: Little, Brown, 1995:396.

Rigsby DC, Macones GA, Driscoll DA. Risk factors for rapid repeat pregnancy among adolescent mother: a review of the literature. *J Pediatr Adolesc Gynecol* 1998;11: 115.

Trad PV. Mental health of adolescent mothers. *J Am Acad Child Adolesc Psychiatry* 1995:34:130.

Grandparents as Parents

People other than parents are increasingly being called on to raise children. Usually the parents are unable to care for their children because of incarceration, illness, drug abuse, suicide, murder, or accidental death. In the great majority of these families, drugs and alcohol are the underlying cause. Black grandparents more frequently raise grandchildren than other races. Awareness of the difficulties these grandparents face will enable family physicians to provide better health care to both the grandparents and the grandchildren.

MEDICAL CONCERNS

Children in the care of grandparents may have suffered medical neglect. The grandparents should try to determine where the child received previous medical care, especially for immunization records. If the grandparents are in contact with a parent, they should obtain a medical release. If the child protective services is involved, they may be able to facilitate obtaining medical records. The physician should be especially thorough in the physical examination, as a full history is rarely available. Signs of physical abuse should be documented. Many of these children suffer from mental disorders such as depression and attention deficit hyperactivity disorder. These conditions may be especially difficult to diagnose when the child is coping with the move to the grandparents' home. Serial evaluations may be necessary. In general, these children should be seen more frequently soon after moving to their new home.

The grandparents themselves may need additional medical care. Financial concerns may force a return to work, or sleepless nights may cause physical stress. Anxiety and depression may improve with relaxation, counseling, or medication.

LEGAL CONCERNS

Many grandparents care for their grandchildren through no legal arrangement. They simply started caring for the children when the parents did not. Unfortunately, in this situation the parents retain legal custody of the child and are the only ones who can give medical and legal consent for them. If the parents are unable or unwilling to meet this responsibility, the grandparents will need to take legal steps to obtain guardianship. This process may incur legal fees but is necessary if the grandparents will need to make medical decisions for the child. In general, these grandparents are eligible for government assistance to support these children if the parent does not.

Some children are placed with grandparents through the child protective system. In this case the court retains legal custody. These "foster" grandparents often may consent for routine medical care, such as office visits, but the agency is involved in more serious situations, such as surgical consent.

Some grandparents adopt the grandchildren. In this case the grandparent in effect becomes the parent and so has all the legal and financial responsibility of a biologic parent.

Overall the legal concerns of these families can be quite confusing. Grandparents often benefit from keeping a detailed log of their interactions with the parents, courts, medical providers, and schools. In this way they have credible information when they interact with the legal system.

GRIEVING

The family where the grandparents are raising the grandchildren is often grieving multiple losses. The parents may have died or been incarcerated. The grandparents may feel their own inadequacy may have led to their child's problems, even if this is not correct. The children may feel that their misbehavior may have caused their parents to be unable to care for them.

FINANCIAL CONCERNS

Grandparents vary widely in their financial ability to care for their grandchildren. For some on a fixed income, raising one or more grandchildren may be a large financial burden. Retired grandparents may need to return to the workforce to support their new families. Retirement communities may not allow children or apartments may not have adequate space.

SOCIAL INTERACTIONS

The social interactions of the grandparents may change fundamentally with the addition of the new children. The grandparents may relate to each other differently with the children in the home. Often the grandfather may have had little interaction with his own young children, so these children may be a new experience for him. One parent may have mixed feelings about taking in the children, or the children may be from another relationship. The parents may make deliberate attempts to disrupt the family. Grandparents may also have difficulty relating to peers who may have more free time and grandparents may regret the loss of their retirement.

EDUCATION

Many of the children raised by grandparents have special educational needs. Young children may benefit from early intervention programs. School-aged children may need an individual educational plan. Grandparents may need to learn to be effective advocates for the children. In their favor, many of these children lacked early educational opportunities, and so they may make rapid progress in a more ideal setting. Some studies have shown that children raised by grandparents had fewer behavioral problems in school than children raised by a single biologic parent (Solomon).

REFERENCES

De Toledo S, Brown DE. Grandparents as parents: a survival guide for raising a second family. New York: Guilford Press, 1995.

Fuller-Thomson E, Minkler M, Driver D. A profile of grandparents raising grandchildren in the United States. *Gerontologist* 1997;37:406.

Solomon JC, Marx J. "To grandmother's house we go": health and school adjustment of children raised solely by grandparents. *Gerontologist* 1995;35:386.

Patient Resources

AARP Grandparent Information Center
AARP Headquarters
601 E St., N.W.
Washington, DC 20049
202-434-2296

Grandparents as Parents
PO Box 964
Lakewood, CA 90714
310-924-3996

Grandparents United for Children's Rights
137 Larkin St.
Madison, WI 53705
608-238-8751

CHAPTER 11

. . . .

Office Emergencies

DEALING WITH OFFICE EMERGENCIES

Fortunately, pediatric office emergencies are not common. Yet they do occur, and family physicians need to be prepared for them. Individual practices vary in the frequency of pediatric office emergencies, depending on the availability of emergency services in the community, the severity of pediatric illness treated in the practice, and the practice triage protocols. Anticipated ambulance response times vary, depending on weather, traffic, and practice location.

Equipment

Preparedness for emergencies begins with equipping the office for emergencies. As most pediatric emergencies involve the respiratory system this equipment has the highest priority. Table 11.1 lists suggested office supplies. If the physician is not proficient in intubation, intubation equipment is not needed. Children can generally be well ventilated with a bag-valve mask, especially if one provider is solely responsible for keeping the mask well positioned during ventilation. Table 11.2 lists suggested emergency medications and fluids. The need for particular equipment and medications will vary with the types of patients seen in the office as well as anticipated emergency medical response times and capabilities.

The equipment should be well labeled and organized, such as in a fishing tackle box, athletic bag with multiple compartments, or a crash cart. All providers, including physicians, should be aware of the organization of the equipment, and it should be kept in an easily accessible location. Dosage charts should be stored with the emergency equipment. The Broslow Tape lists pediatric medication doses and equipment sizes based on the child's length or weight. Its small size and convenient organization make this an ideal reference. Algorithms for management of common emergencies are also helpful. These algorithms are available in the Pediatric Advance Life Support Textbook or in standard pediatric references such as the Harriet Lane Handbook.

Training

Within the office, providers need to be adequately trained to handle emergencies. This training can be obtained through the American Heart Association Basic Life Support and Pediatric Advanced Life Support Courses. Staff should be trained in appropriate phone triage for potential emergencies. They should also be aware of signs of a potential emergency in the waiting room.

All staff should be aware of the protocol for activating the emergency medical system.

Practice

Once the training and equipment are obtained, practice sessions or "Mock codes" should be performed regularly. These allow the staff to practice with the equipment and emphasize the importance of emergency preparedness.

T ABLE 11.1. Suggested emergency equipment for physician offices

Airway Management
Nasal cannulas—infant, child, and adult sizes 1–3
Oral airways—0–5
Oxygen masks—infant, child, adult
Oxygen source with flowmeter (to deliver >15 mL/min)
Self-initiating bag-valve—mask resuscitators, including reservoir—infant, child, adult
Suction catheters—Yanksauer, 8F, 10F, 14F
Suction—wall or machine
Optional for intubation
    Endotracheal tubes, uncuffed sizes 2.5–6.0 and cuffed 6.0–8.0
    Laryngoscope batteries and bulbs
    Laryngoscope handle with Miller or Wishipple blades—0, 1, 2, 3
    Magill forceps—pediatric and adult
    Stylets—pediatric and adult sizes for endotracheal tubes
Fluid Management
Intraosseous needles—15 and 18 gauge
Intravenous catheters—14–24 gauge
Isotonic fluids (normal saline or lactated Ringer's solution)
IV boards, tape, alcohol swabs, tourniquet
Pediatric drip chambers and tubing
Optional: over-guidewire catheters—3F, 4F, 5F
Miscellaneous Equipment
Blood pressure cuffs—infant, child, adult
Cardiac arrest board
Feeding tubes—3F, 5F
Foley urine catheters—8F, 10F
Nasogastric tubes—10F, 14F
Sphygmomanometer
Optional Equipment
Noninvasive blood pressure monitor
Portable ECG monitor/defibrillator
Pulse oximeter

Used with permission from Pediatric Advanced Life Support. Dallas, TX: American Heart Association, 1997.

T ABLE 11.2.   Emergency medications and fluids

Normal saline or lactated Ringer's solution
Albuterol (Ventolin) (0.5%) for inhalation
Epinephrine 1:1,000 and 1:10,000 concentration
D50 (dilute 1:1 with sterile water before using)
Atropine (0.1 mg/mL)
Lorazepam (Ativan) (2 mg/mL)
Sterile water
Parenteral corticosteroid (i.e., methylprednisolone [Solumedrol] or dexamethasone [Decadron])
Parenteral antibiotic (i.e., ceftriaxone [Rocephin])

Physician Resources

American Heart Association. www.americanheart.org Provides links to local chapters.

Armstrong Medical. 800-323-4220. Broslow Tapes, airway supplies,

Repro-Med. 800-637-9990. Manufacturer of the Res-Q-Vac portable suction ($50).

REFERENCES

Chameides L, Hazinski MF, eds. *Pediatric Advanced Life Support.* Dallas, TX: American Heart Association, 1997.

Flores G, Weinstock DJ. The preparedness of pediatricians for emergencies in the office. What is broken, should we care, how can we fix it? *Arch Pediatr Adolesc Med* 1996;150:249.

Schumann AJ. Be prepared: equipping your office for medical emergencies. *Contemp Pediatr* 1996;13(7):27–43.

Siberry GK, Ianonne R, eds. *The Harriet Lane handbook*, 15th ed. St Louis, MO: Mosby, 2000.

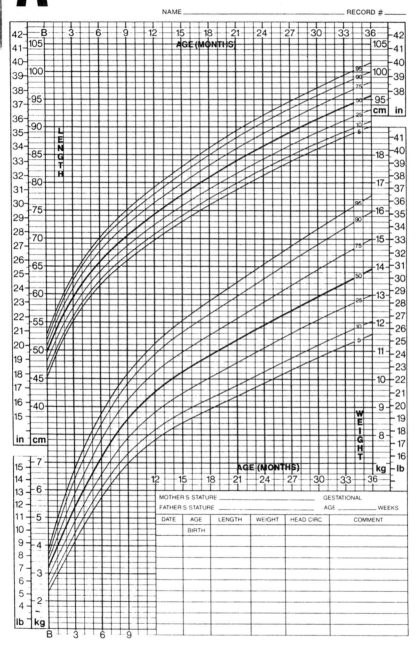

FIGURE 1. National Center for Health Statistics percentiles of physical growth in girls from birth to 36 months of age. (Copyright 1982 Ross Laboratories, Columbus, OH 43216. Adapted from Hamill PVV, Drizd TA, Johnson CL, et al. Physical growth: National Center for Health Statistics percentiles. *Am J Clin Nutr* 1979;32:607. Data from the Fels Research Institute, Wright State University School of Medicine, Yellow Springs, OH.)

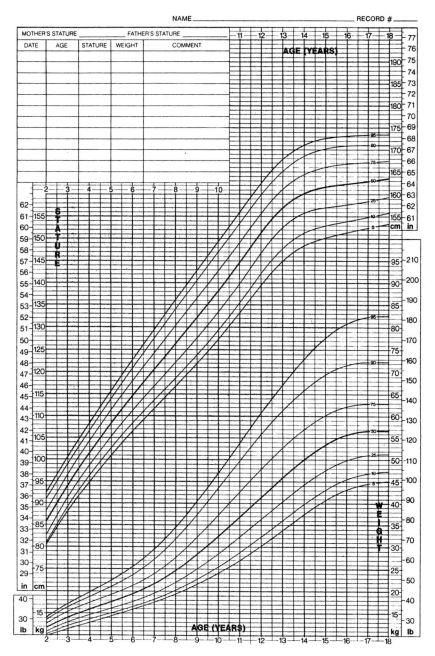

FIGURE 2. National Center for Health Statistics percentiles of physical growth in girls 2 to 18 years of age. (Copyright 1982 Ross Laboratories, Columbus, OH 43216. Adapted from Hamill PVV, Drizd TA, Johnson CL, et al. Physical growth: National Center for Health Statistics percentiles. *Am J Clin Nutr* 1979;32:607. Data from the National Center for Health Statistics, Hyattsville, MD.)

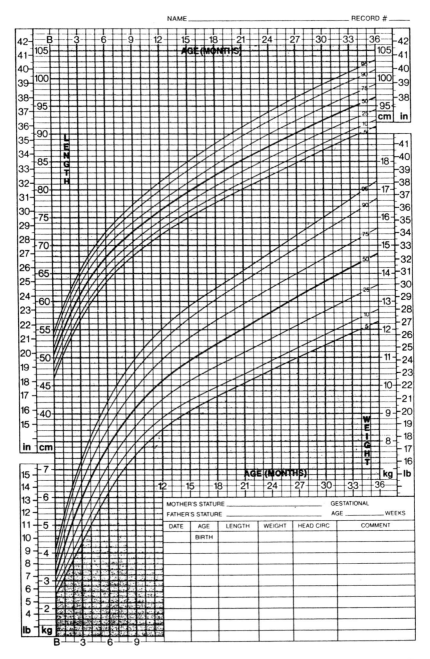

FIGURE 3. National Center for Health Statistics percentiles of physical growth in boys from birth to 36 months of age. (Copyright 1982 Ross Laboratories, Columbus, OH 43216. Adapted from Hamill PVV, Drizd TA, Johnson CL, et al. Physical growth: National Center for Health Statistics percentiles. *Am J Clin Nutr* 1979;32:607. Data from the Fels Research Institute, Wright State University School of Medicine, Yellow Springs, OH.)

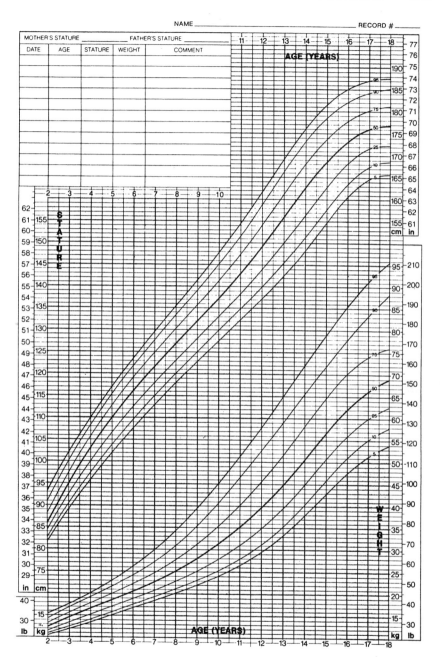

FIGURE 4. National Center for Health Statistics percentiles of physical growth in boys 2 to 18 years of age. (Copyright 1982 Ross Laboratories, Columbus, OH 43216. Adapted from Hamill PVV, Drizd TA, Johnson CL, et al. Physical growth: National Center for Health Statistics percentiles. *Am J Clin Nutr* 1979;32:607. Data from the National Center for Health Statistics, Hyattsville, MD.)

	SOCIAL	SELF-HELP	GROSS MOTOR	FINE MOTOR	LANGUAGE	
5-0 yrs.	Shows leadership among children	Goes to the toilet without help	Swings on swing, pumping by self	Prints first name (four letters)	Tells meaning of familiar words	**5-0** yrs.
4-6	Follows simple game rules in board games or card games	Usually looks both ways before crossing street	Skips or makes running "broad jumps"	Draws a person that has at least three parts - head, eyes, nose, mouth, etc.	Reads a few letters (five+)	**4-6**
4-0 yrs.	Protective toward younger children	Buttons one or more buttons	Hops around on one foot, without support	Draws recognizable pictures	Follows a series of three simple instructions	**4-0** yrs.
		Dresses and undresses without help, except for tying shoelaces			Understands concepts - size, number, shape	
3-6	Plays cooperatively, with minimum conflict and supervision	Washes face without help	Hops on one foot, without support	Cuts across paper with small scissors	Counts five or more objects when asked "How many?"	**3-6**
				Draws or copies a complete circle	Identifies four colors correctly	
3-0 yrs.	Gives directions to other children	Toilet trained	Rides around on a tricycle, using pedals		Combines sentences with the words "and," "or," or "but"	**3-0** yrs.
		Dresses self with help	Walks up and down stairs ⅄ one foot per step	Cuts with small scissors		
2-6	Plays a role in "pretend" games - mom-dad, teacher, space pilot	Washes and dries hands	Stands on one foot without support	Draws or copies vertical (│) lines	Understands four prepositions - in, on, under, beside	**2-6**
	Plays with other children - cars, dolls, building				Talks clearly - is understandable most of the time	
	"Helps" with simple household tasks	Opens door by turning knob	Climbs on play equipment - ladders, slides	Scribbles with circular motion	Talks in two-three word phrases or sentences	

Age	Social	Self-help / Feeding	Gross Motor	Fine Motor	Language / Hearing
2-0 yrs.	Usually responds to correction - stops; Shows sympathy to other children, tries to comfort them	Takes off open coat or shirt without help; Eats with spoon, spilling little	Walks up and down stairs alone; Runs well, seldom falls	Turns pages of picture books, one at a time; Builds towers of four or more blocks	Follows two-part instructions; Uses at least ten words
18 mos.	Sometimes says "No" when interfered with; Greets people with "Hi" or similar	Eats with fork; Insists on doing things by self such as feeding	Kicks a ball forward; Runs	Scribbles with crayon; Stacks two or more blocks	Follows simple instructions; Asks for food or drink with words; Talks in single words
12 mos.	Gives kisses or hugs; Wants stuffed animal, doll or blanket in bed; Plays patty-cake	Feeds self with spoon; Lifts cup to mouth and drinks; Picks up a spoon by the handle	Walks without help; Stands without support; Walks around furniture or crib while holding on	Picks up two small toys in one hand; Picks up small objects - precise thumb and finger grasp	Uses one or two words as names of things or actions; Understands words like "No," "Stop," or "All gone"; Word sounds - says "Ma-ma" or "Da-da" as name for parent
9 mos.	Plays social games, peek-a-boo, bye-bye; Pushes things away he/she doesn't want		Crawls around on hands and knees; Sits alone ... steady, without support	Picks up object with thumb and finger grasp	Wide range of vocalizations (vowel sounds, consonant-vowel combinations)
6 mos.	Reaches for familiar persons; Distinguishes mother from others	Feeds self cracker; Comforts self with thumb or pacifier	Rolls over from back to stomach; Turns around when lying on stomach	Transfers toy from one hand to the other; Picks up toy with one hand	Responds to name - turns and looks; Vocalizes spontaneously, social
Birth	Social smile	Reacts to sight of bottle or breast	Lifts head and chest when lying on stomach	Looks at and reaches for faces and toys	Reacts to voices; Vocalizes, coos, chuckles

FIGURE 5. Child Development in the first 5 years.

TABLE A.1. Recommended childhood immunization schedule, United States—January 2000 to December 2000

Age Vaccine	Birth	1 mo	2 mos	4 mos	6 mos	12 mos	15 mos	18 mos	24 mos	4–6 yrs	11–12 yrs	14–16 yrs
Hepatitis B†	Hep B →	Hep B →				Hep B					Hep	
			Hep B →									
Diphtheria, Tetanus, Pertussis‡			DTaP	DTaP	DTaP		DTaP† →			DTaP	Td →	Td →
Haemophilus influenzae Type b§			Hib	Hib	Hib	Hib →	Hib →					
Polio‖			IPV	IPV	IPV →	IPV →	IPV →			IPV‖		
Measles, Mumps, Rubella¶						MMR →	MMR →			MMR¶	MMR¶	
Varicella#						Var →	Var →				Var¶	
Hepatitis A**									← Hep A**, in selected areas →			

Note: On October 22, 1999, the Advisory Committee on Immunization Practices (ACIP) recommended that Rotashield (RRV-TV), the only U.S.-licensed rotavirus vaccine, no longer can be used in the United States (MMWR, Volume 48, Number 43, November 5, 1999). Parents should be reassured that their children who received rotavirus vaccine before July are not at increased risk for intussusception now.

This schedule has been approved by the ACIP, the American Academy of Pediatrics (AAP) and the American Academy of Family Physicians (AAFP). It indicates the recommended ages for routine administration of currently licensed childhood vaccines as of November 1, 1999. Licensed combination vaccines may be used whenever any components of the combination are indicated and its other components are not contraindicated. Providers should consult the manufacturers' package inserts for detailed recommendations.

Vaccines are listed under routinely recommended ages. Clear bars indicate range of recommended ages for immunization. Any dose not given at the recommended age should be given as a "catch-up" immunization at any subsequent visit when indicated and feasible. Shaded ovals indicate vaccines to be given if previously recommended doses were missed or given earlier than the recommended minimum age.

†Infants born to hepatitis B surface antigen (HBsAg)-negative mothers should receive the first dose of hepatitis B (Hep B) vaccine by age two months. The second dose should be given at least one month after the first dose. The third dose should be administered at least four months after the first dose and at least two months after the second dose, but not before six months of age for infants. Infants born to HBsAg-positive mothers should receive hepatitis B vaccine and 0.5 mL hepatitis B immune globulin (HBIG) within 12 hours of birth at separate sites. The second dose is recommended at one to two months of age and the third dose at 6 months of age. Infants born to mothers whose HBsAg status is unknown should receive hepatitis B vaccine within 12 hours of birth. Maternal blood should be drawn at the time of delivery to determine the mother's HBsAg status; if the HBsAg test is positive, the infant should receive HBIG as soon as possible (no later than 1 week of age). All children and adolescents (through 18 years of age) who have not been immunized against hepatitis B may begin the series during any visit. Special efforts should be made to immunize children who were born in or whose parents were born in areas of the world with moderate or high endemicity of hepatitis B virus infection.

‡The fourth dose of diphtheria and tetanus toxoids and acellular pertussis vaccine (DTaP) may be administered as early as 12 months of age, provided 6 months has elapsed since the third dose and if the child is unlikely to return at age 15 to 18 months. Tetanus and diphtheria toxoids (Td) immunization is recommended at 11 to 12 years of age if at least 5 years has elapsed since the last dose of DTP, DTaP, or DT. Subsequent routine Td boosters are recommended every 10 years.

§Three *Haemophilus influenza* type b (Hib) conjugate vaccines are licensed for infant use. If PRP-OMP (PedvaxHIB and COMVAX) is administered at 2 and 4 months of age, a dose at 6 months is not required. Because clinical studies in infants have demonstrated that using some combination products may induce a lower immune response to the Hib vaccine component, DTaP/Hib combination products should not be used for primary immunization in infants at 2, 4, or 6 months of age, unless it is approved by the US Food and Drug Administration for these ages.

||To eliminate the risk of vaccine-associated paralytic polio (VAPP), an all-inactivated poliovirus vaccine (IPV) schedule is now recommended for routine childhood polio vaccination in the United States. All children should receive four doses of IPV at 2 months, 4 months, 6 to 18 months, and 4 to 6 years. Oral poliovirus vaccine (OPV), if available, may be used only for the following special circumstances: (1) mass vaccination campaigns to control outbreaks of paralytic polio; (2) unvaccinated children who will be traveling in less than 4 weeks to areas where polio is endemic or epidemic; (3) children of parents who do not accept the recommended number of vaccine injections. These children may receive OPV only for the third or fourth dose, or both; in this situation, health care providers should administer OPV only after discussing the risk for VAPP with parents or caregivers; (4) during the transition to an all-IPV schedule, recommendations for the use of remaining OPV supplies in physicians' offices and clinics have been issued by the AAP (see *Pediatrics*, December 1999).

¶The second dose of measles-mumps-rubella (MMR) vaccine is recommended routinely at 4 to 6 years of age but may be administered during any visit, provided at least 4 weeks has elapsed since receipt of the first dose and that both doses are administered beginning at or after 12 months of age. Those who have not previously received the second dose should complete the schedule by the 11- to 12-year-old visit.

#Varicella (Var) vaccine is recommended at any visit on or after the first birthday for susceptible children, i.e., those who lack a reliable history of chickenpox (as judged by a health care provider) and who have not been immunized. Susceptible persons 13 years of age or older should receive two doses, given at least 4 weeks apart.

**Hepatitis A (Hep A) is shaded to indicate its recommended use in selected states and/or regions; consult your local public health authority. (Also see *MMWR* October 1, 1999;48(RR-12):1–37.)

This schedule is provided by the American Academy of Family Physicians only as an assistance for physicians making clinical decisions regarding the care of their patients. As such, they cannot substitute for the individual judgment brought to each clinical situation by the patient's family physician. As with all clinical reference resources, they reflect the best understanding of the science of medicine at the time of publication, but they should be used with the clear understanding that continued research may result in new knowledge and recommendations.

T ABLE A.2.   Minimal interval between vaccine doses for use when immunization is behind schedule*

Vaccine Type	Minimal Interval Between Dose 1 and 2	Minimal Interval Between Dose 2 and 3	Minimal Interval Between Dose 3 and 4
Hepatitis B	1 month	2 months†	
DTP/DTaP (DT)‡	4 weeks	4 weeks	6 months
Hib (primary series)			
HbOC	1 month	1 month	2 months and age at least 12 months
PRP-T	1 month	1 month	2 months and age at least 12 months
PRP-OMP	1 month	2 months and age at least 12 months	
Poliovirus	4 weeks	4 weeks	No earlier than 4 years
MMR‖	1 month‖		

Abbreviations: DTP/DTaP (DT), diphtheria and tetanus toxoids and whole-cell pertussis vaccine/diphtheria and tetanus toxoids and acellular pertussis vaccine (diphtheria and tetanus toxoids vaccine); Hib, *Haemophilus influenzae* type b conjugate vaccine; HbOC, oligosaccharides conjugated to diphtheria CRM_{197} toxin protein; PRP-T, polyribosylribitol phosphate polysaccharide conjugated to tetanus toxoid; PRP-OMP, polyribosylribitol phosphate polysaccharide conjugated to a meningococcal outer membrane protein; MMR, measles-mumps-rubella vaccine.

*The minimal acceptable intervals may not correspond with the optimal recommended ages and intervals for vaccination.

†This final dose of hepatitis B vaccine is recommended at least 4 months after the first dose and no earlier than 6 months of age.

‡The total number of doses of diphtheria and tetanus toxoids should not exceed six each before the seventh birthday.

‖Although the age for measles vaccination may be as young as six months in outbreak areas where cases are occurring in children less than one year of age, children initially vaccinated before the first birthday should be revaccinated at 12 to 15 months of age and an additional dose of vaccine should be administered at the time of school entry or according to local policy.

Adapted from *Epidemiology and prevention of vaccine-preventable deceases.* 5th ed. Atlanta: Centers for Disease Control and Prevention, 1999.

TABLE A.3. Acetaminophen dosing

Weight (pounds)	Age	Concentrated Drops, 80 mg/0.8 mL	Suspension or Elixir, 160 mg/5 mL	Chewable, 80 mg/tablet
6–11	0–3 months	½ dropper (0.4 mL)		
12–17	4–11 months	1 dropper (0.8 mL)		
18–23	12–24 months		½ teaspoon (2.5 mL)	
			¾ teaspoon	
24–35	2–3 years		1 teaspoon (5 mL)	2 tablets
36–47	4–5 years		1½ teaspoons (7.5 mL)	3 tablets
48–59	6–8 years		2 teaspoons (10 mL)	4 tablets
60–71	9–10 years			5 tablets
72–95	11–12 years	—		6 tablets

Based on dosage of 10–15 mg/kg/dose.

Use weight-based dosing when the weight is available.

Dose every 4–6 hours.

T ABLE A.4. Ibuprofen dosing

Weight (pounds)	Age	Concentrated Drops, 40 mg/mL	Suspension, 100 mg/5 mL	Chewable Tablets, 50 mg	Chewable Tablets/Caplets, 100 mg
12–17	6–11 months	1 dropper (1.25 mL)			
18–23	12–23 months	1½ dropper (1.9 mL)			
24–35	2–3 years		1 teaspoon (5 mL)		
36–47	4–5 years		1½ teaspoons (7.5 mL)	3 tablets	
48–59	6–8 years		2 teaspoons (10 mL)	4 tablets	2 tablets/caplets
60–71	9–10 years		2½ teaspoons (12.5 mL)	5 tablets	2.5 tablets/caplets
72–95	11 years		3 teaspoons (15 mL)	6 tablets	3 tablets/caplets

Based on dosage of 5–10 mg/kg/dose.
Use weight-based dosing when the weight is available.
Dose every 6–8 hours.

SUBJECT INDEX

Note: Page numbers in italics indicate figures; page numbers followed by *t* indicate tables.

A

Abscess, breast, 5
Accident prevention, teenagers, 70
Acetaminophen dosage, 248*t*
Acne, 72, 73*t*
Adolescents
  See also Well-child visits.
  accident prevention, 70
  anorexia and bulimia, 212-222
  depression, 222-227
  diabetes mellitus, 185
  HIV infection, 192
  knee pain, 114
  teenage mothers, 232-234
Adoption, grandparents as parents, 234-235
Advocacy, foster children, 231
Alarms, enuresis, 124, 125
Alcohol use, teenagers, 71
Algorithms
  head malformation, 29
  hematuria, 127
  office emergencies, 237
  proteinuria, 129
  urinary tract infection, 134
Allergens
  asthma, 157, 158
  formula intolerance, 10-11
  solid foods, 32-33
Alport's syndrome, 126, 128
Amblyopia, 58
Anorexia and bulimia, 212-222
  differential diagnosis, 213, 219, 218*t*
  family history, 213
  follow-up, 220
  history, 212-213
  laboratory evaluation, 213, 218*t*
  management, 219, 221*t*
  parent and patient resources, 222
  physical examination, 213, 214-217*t*
  professional resources, 222
  references, 220-222
  referral, 219, 220*t*
  social history, 213
Antiretroviral therapy, HIV infection,
    189-190
Apnea, premature infant, 196, 197*t*
Arthritis, septic, hip problems, 118-119
Asthma, 157-180
  diagnosis, 158, 158*t*
  exacerbations, 159, 165, *174-175*
  exercise-induced, 165
  family history, 157
  follow-up, 180
  history of present illness, 157
  laboratory testing, 158
  management, 159, *164-167*, 170-173*t*

medical history, 157
medication delivery, 165, 178, *176-177*
monitoring, 159, *160-163*, 164*t*
parent resources, 180
patient education, 178-179, *178-179*
physical examination, 158
references, 180
referral, 180
social history, 157
Athletic participation, 76-84
  clearance, 76-77, 80-83*t*
  history, 76, 77
  laboratory evaluation, 76
  medical/legal considerations, 78
  physical examination, 76, 78*t*
  references, 78
Attention-deficit hyperactivity disorder,
    203-212
  books for children, 212
  chief complaint, 203
  diagnosis, 207
  differential diagnosis, 206*t*
  family history, 203
  follow-up, 210-211, 210*t*
  grandparents as parents, 234
  history of present illness, 203, 204-205*t*
  laboratory evaluation, 207
  management, 207, 210
  medication, 208-209*t*
  parent resources, 211
  physical examination, 207
  physician resources, 211
  references, 211-212
  referral, 211
  social history, 203

B

Barolow maneuver, 23, *23*
Bed-wetting, 123-125
  alarms, 125
  chief complaint, 123
  differential diagnosis, 124
  family history, 123
  history of present illness, 123
  laboratory evaluation, 124
  medical history, 123
  patient education, 125
  physical examination, 123
  references, 125
  referral, 125
  social history, 123
  treatment, 124, 124-125*t*
Behavior, in mental retardation, 187
Behavioral management
  attention-deficit hyperactivity disorder, 207
  bed-wetting, 124, 124*t*